Gut Instincts

Harnessing the Power of Microbial Health

A short introduction by The HealthSpan Institute

Contents

Chapter 4:
The Gut-Brain Connection

Chapter 5:
Gut Microbiome and Physical Health

Chapter 6:
Diet and Your Microbiome

Chapter 7:
Lifestyle and Microbial Health

Chapter 8:
Rebalancing Your Microbiome

Chapter 9:
Innovations in Microbiome Research

Chapter 10:
Practical Strategies for Everyday Wellness

Chapter 11:
The Future of Microbiome Health

Chapter 12: Conclusion

Chapter 1: Introduction

Exploring the Concept of Gut Instincts

The term "gut instincts" often conjures images of a deep-seated, intuitive knowing, an unspoken wisdom that seems to arise from the very core of our being. While this metaphorical understanding has its roots in psychological and philosophical realms, recent scientific discoveries have added a fascinating layer to this concept, revealing a literal truth underlying this age-old idiom. The exploration of the gut microbiome, an intricate and diverse ecosystem of microorganisms residing in our digestive tract, has opened new frontiers in understanding the intricate connection between our gut health and overall well-being. This chapter delves into the multifaceted nature of gut instincts, bridging the gap between metaphorical intuition and the burgeoning field of microbiome research.

Traditionally, gut instincts have been viewed as the human body's primal response mechanism, guiding decisions in the absence of rational thought. It is the sensation that nudges us towards a certain path or warns us against potential danger, often without a clear rationale. Philosophers and psychologists have long debated the origins and validity of these instincts, with some considering them as remnants of our evolutionary past, while others view them as an integral part of human cognition. However, with the advent of modern science, particularly in the realm of microbiology and neurogastroenterology, the concept of gut instincts has transcended its metaphorical boundaries, revealing a complex interplay between our gut health and our mental and emotional states.

The human gut microbiome is a complex and dynamic ecosystem, comprising bacteria, fungi, viruses, and other microorganisms. These microbial communities play a crucial role in various physiological processes, including digestion, immune function, and even the production of neurotransmitters. Interestingly, research has shown that the gut microbiome can influence our mood, preferences, and behavior, suggesting a biological basis for the phenomenon of gut instincts. The gut-brain axis, a bidirectional communication network linking the enteric nervous system in the gut with the central nervous system, serves as a conduit for this interaction, allowing the gut microbiome to send signals directly to the brain.

This revelation has profound implications for our understanding of human psychology and behavior. The idea that our gut can "communicate" with our brain and potentially influence our decisions adds a tangible dimension to the concept of gut instincts. For instance, cravings for certain foods may not just be a matter of personal taste but could also be influenced by the needs or imbalances of our gut microbiota. Similarly, the "butterflies" in the stomach often experienced in stressful situations could be indicative of the microbiome's response to psychological stress.

Moreover, the gut microbiome's impact on mental health has opened new avenues in treating disorders such as anxiety and depression. The concept of "psychobiotics" – probiotics that can potentially improve mental health by influencing the gut-brain axis – is an emerging field of research, offering hope for new, holistic approaches to mental health care. This intertwining of physical and mental health underscores the importance of maintaining a healthy gut microbiome for overall well-being.

Understanding and nurturing our gut microbiome thus becomes a critical aspect of listening to and interpreting our gut instincts. Diet, lifestyle, stress management, and environmental factors all play significant roles in shaping the composition and health of our gut microbiota. By fostering a diverse and balanced gut ecosystem, we may enhance our ability to tap into this ancient form of wisdom, making more informed and health-conscious decisions.

As we delve deeper into the mysteries of the gut microbiome, the literal and metaphorical interpretations of gut instincts continue to converge. What was once considered a mere figure of speech is now being acknowledged as a complex, bidirectional relationship between our gut and our brain. This newfound understanding not only enriches our perception of human intuition but also highlights the remarkable sophistication of our body's internal systems. The exploration of the gut microbiome is not just a scientific endeavor; it is a journey towards understanding the profound wisdom that resides within us, waiting to be acknowledged and harnessed for our health and happiness.

In conclusion, the concept of gut instincts is an intricate tapestry woven from threads of ancient wisdom, psychological theory, and modern scientific research. As we stand at the crossroads of these diverse fields, the exploration of our gut microbiome offers a unique perspective, shedding light on the literal and figurative significance of listening to our gut. By embracing this holistic view, we open ourselves to a deeper understanding of our bodies, our minds, and the invisible yet powerful forces that guide our health and decisions. Gut instincts, once a metaphor for intuition, now emerge as a tangible indicator of our body's inner workings, reminding us of the intricate connection between our physical and mental selves.

Overview of the Gut Microbiome

In recent years, the gut microbiome has emerged as a key player in human health, sparking a revolution in our understanding of the human body. This complex community of microorganisms residing in our digestive tract is not merely a passive collection of bacteria, but an active and dynamic participant in our health and well-being. This chapter provides an overview of the gut microbiome, exploring its composition, functions, and the profound impact it has on our lives.

The gut microbiome is a diverse ecosystem, hosting trillions of microorganisms, including bacteria, viruses, fungi, and protozoa. Each individual's microbiome is unique, shaped by a variety of factors such as genetics, diet, lifestyle, and environmental exposures. The development of this microbiome begins at birth and evolves throughout life, reflecting changes in our environment and lifestyle. The composition of this microbial community is critical; a balanced microbiome is associated with good health, while imbalances have been linked to numerous diseases.

One of the key functions of the gut microbiome is aiding in digestion. It helps in breaking down complex carbohydrates, fibers, and proteins, some of which are indigestible by human enzymes. These processes not only provide us with essential nutrients but also produce short-chain fatty acids (SCFAs) like butyrate, propionate, and acetate. SCFAs play crucial roles in maintaining gut health, regulating metabolism, and even modulating immune responses. This highlights the gut microbiome's vital role in nutrition and metabolic health.

Moreover, the gut microbiome forms an integral part of the body's immune system. It helps in distinguishing between harmful and benign substances and trains the immune system to respond appropriately. A healthy microbiome acts as a barrier against pathogens, preventing them from colonizing the gut. Imbalances in the microbiome, known as dysbiosis, have been linked to autoimmune diseases, allergies, and even certain types of cancer. This underscores the microbiome's role in maintaining immune homeostasis and its potential in preventing and treating disease.

The concept of the gut-brain axis further illustrates the extensive influence of the gut microbiome. This bidirectional communication system between the gut and the brain implicates the microbiome in various aspects of neurological and psychological health. Research has shown that changes in the gut microbiome can affect mood, behavior, and cognitive functions. The gut microbiome produces various neurotransmitters and signaling molecules, suggesting a direct pathway through which it can influence brain function. This connection opens new pathways for understanding and treating neurological and psychiatric disorders.

The gut microbiome's interaction with other body systems, such as the endocrine and cardiovascular systems, further demonstrates its multifaceted role. For instance, certain gut bacteria can influence hormone production, impacting everything from stress responses to reproductive health. Similarly, there is growing evidence linking gut microbiota composition to heart health, including the regulation of blood pressure and cholesterol levels.

Diet plays a crucial role in shaping the gut microbiome. Dietary patterns rich in diverse plant-based foods tend to promote a more diverse and stable microbiome, which is associated with better health outcomes. Conversely, diets high in processed foods, sugar, and unhealthy fats can lead to a less diverse microbiome, contributing to various health issues. This relationship between diet and the microbiome offers a powerful tool for improving health through dietary interventions.

The rapidly evolving field of microbiome research continues to uncover the vast potential of the gut microbiome in health and disease. Innovations in sequencing technologies and computational biology have allowed for more in-depth analysis of the microbiome, leading to a better understanding of its complexity and function. This research is not only enhancing our understanding of human biology but is also paving the way for novel therapeutic strategies, ranging from probiotics and prebiotics to fecal microbiota transplantation.

In conclusion, the gut microbiome is a complex and dynamic entity that plays a crucial role in various aspects of human health. Its influence extends far beyond the digestive tract, impacting immune function, brain health, metabolic processes, and much more. As we continue to unravel the mysteries of the gut microbiome, it becomes increasingly clear that maintaining a healthy and balanced microbiome is essential for overall health and well-being. This burgeoning field holds great promise for the future of medicine and health care, offering new insights and approaches to preventing and treating a wide range of conditions. The gut microbiome, once a neglected aspect of human biology, now stands at the forefront of a new era in health and disease understanding.

The Importance of Microbial Health

The exploration of the human microbiome, particularly the diverse ecosystem of microorganisms residing in our gut, has fundamentally altered our understanding of health and disease. Microbial health, which refers to the balance and function of these microorganisms, is now recognized as a crucial factor in our overall well-being. This essay delves into the various dimensions of microbial health, underscoring its significance in human physiology, disease prevention, and potential therapeutic applications.

Microbial health primarily hinges on the diversity and balance of the microbiota within our bodies. A diverse microbiome is typically a sign of good health, as it indicates a wide range of functional capabilities and resilience against pathogenic invasions. The gut microbiome, comprising bacteria, fungi, viruses, and other microorganisms, plays a vital role in numerous bodily functions. It is not only instrumental in digestion and nutrient absorption but also significantly influences the immune system, mental health, and even the risk of chronic diseases.

One of the most crucial functions of a healthy microbiome is its role in the development and maintenance of the immune system. A balanced gut microbiome educates the immune system, helping it distinguish between harmless and harmful pathogens. This interaction is pivotal in preventing autoimmune diseases, where the immune system mistakenly attacks the body's own cells. Moreover, a healthy microbiome produces various substances that strengthen the gut barrier, preventing harmful substances from entering the bloodstream and triggering immune responses.

The impact of microbial health extends to the central nervous system, illustrating the gut-brain axis's significance. Research has uncovered that changes in the gut microbiome can influence mood, behavior, and cognitive functions, with implications for mental health disorders such as depression and anxiety. The gut microbiome communicates with the brain through various pathways, including the vagus nerve, immune signaling, and the production of neurotransmitters and other bioactive molecules. This complex communication network highlights the potential of

modulating the gut microbiome to improve mental health outcomes.

In addition to mental health, microbial health plays a pivotal
role in metabolic processes. The gut microbiome has been linked
to obesity, diabetes, and metabolic syndrome. It influences the
body's metabolism by affecting energy extraction from food, insulin sensitivity, and inflammation – factors that are crucial in the development and progression of metabolic diseases. This connection
offers new perspectives on preventing and managing metabolic
disorders through dietary and lifestyle interventions that promote
a healthy microbiome.

The diversity and balance of the gut microbiome are also
closely tied to dietary habits. Diets rich in fiber, fruits, vegetables,
and fermented foods promote a diverse and healthy microbiome,
while diets high in processed foods, sugars, and unhealthy fats can
lead to dysbiosis, an imbalance in the microbiome associated with
various health issues. Therefore, dietary choices play a pivotal role
in maintaining microbial health and, by extension, overall health.

Emerging research in the field of microbial health is also exploring the therapeutic potential of manipulating the gut microbiome.
Probiotics, prebiotics, and fecal microbiota transplants are being
studied for their potential to restore microbial balance and treat
a range of conditions, from gastrointestinal disorders to autoimmune diseases and beyond. This area of research holds great
promise, offering new, more natural, and holistic approaches to
disease treatment and prevention.

Moreover, the study of microbial health is leading to personalized medicine approaches. Since each individual's microbiome is
unique, treatments and dietary recommendations can be tailored
to their specific microbial composition. This personalized approach
has the potential to revolutionize healthcare, making it more effective and efficient by considering each person's unique microbial
ecosystem.

In conclusion, the importance of microbial health cannot be
overstated. It is a cornerstone of our physical, mental, and meta-

bolic well-being, with far-reaching implications for disease prevention and treatment. As we continue to unravel the complexities of the human microbiome, our approach to health and disease is being transformed. A healthy microbiome is not just about preventing illness; it is about fostering overall health, vitality, and resilience. The future of healthcare will likely see an increased focus on maintaining and restoring microbial health, marking a paradigm shift towards more holistic and personalized medical practices. The burgeoning field of microbial health research is not only enhancing our understanding of the human body but also opening new doors to wellness and longevity.

Chapter 2:
The World Inside Us

A Closer Look at the Human Microbiome

The human microbiome represents one of the most fascinating and complex elements of our biological makeup. It is a thriving community of trillions of microorganisms that inhabit various parts of our body, most notably the gut. This chapter delves into the intricate world of the human microbiome, exploring its composition, functions, and the profound implications it holds for our health and understanding of human biology.

The human microbiome is a diverse ecosystem, comprising bacteria, viruses, fungi, and other microscopic organisms. Each person's microbiome is as unique as their fingerprint, influenced by factors like genetics, birth method, diet, environment, and lifestyle. The most extensive and studied part of the human microbiome is found in the gut, where these microorganisms form a complex and dynamic community. This community is not a mere passenger in our bodies; it plays an active role in our health and well-being.

Understanding the composition of the microbiome is crucial in appreciating its role in our bodies. The gut microbiome, for instance, contains a vast array of bacterial species, each with specific functions. Some bacteria are involved in breaking down food and synthesizing essential nutrients, while others play a critical role in shaping our immune system. The diversity of this microbial population is key to its functionality – a more diverse microbiome is usually associated with better health, as it can perform a broader range of physiological tasks and is more resilient to disturbances.

The functions of the microbiome extend far beyond digestion. The microbiome is integral to the development and function of the immune system, helping to distinguish between friendly and harmful organisms. It also plays a role in the synthesis of vitamins and hormones and even affects our metabolism and energy levels. Recent research has unveiled the microbiome's influence on mental health, contributing to conditions such as anxiety and depression. This vast range of functions underscores the microbiome's importance in maintaining overall health and preventing disease.

The gut microbiome's composition is dynamic and responsive to changes in diet, lifestyle, and environment. Diet, in particular, has a profound impact on the microbiome. A diet rich in diverse plant-based foods can increase microbiome diversity and functionality, whereas a diet high in processed foods can decrease it. This responsiveness offers opportunities for improving health through dietary changes. By understanding how different foods affect the microbiome, individuals can make informed choices to positively influence their health.

The human microbiome also plays a critical role in drug metabolism. The microbiome can affect how drugs are absorbed, metabolized, and excreted from the body, influencing their efficacy and safety. This interaction has significant implications for personalized medicine, suggesting that treatments could be tailored based on an individual's microbiome composition for optimal outcomes.

The microbiome's impact on health is so profound that imbalances in its composition, known as dysbiosis, have been linked to a range of diseases, including inflammatory bowel disease, obesity, diabetes, and even certain types of cancer. Understanding the mechanisms behind these associations is a key area of research, as it could lead to new preventive and therapeutic strategies for these conditions.

The field of microbiome research is rapidly evolving, with new technologies enabling more detailed and comprehensive analysis. Advanced sequencing techniques and computational tools are allowing scientists to explore the microbiome in unprecedented depth, revealing its complexities and interactions with the human body. This research is not only deepening our understanding of human biology but also opening new frontiers in medicine and health care.

In conclusion, the human microbiome is a vital component of our biology, influencing almost every aspect of our health. From digestion and immunity to mental health and drug metabolism, the microbiome plays a pivotal role. Its diversity and dynamism make it a powerful ally in maintaining health and preventing disease. As we continue to explore this fascinating world inside us, we are likely to uncover even more ways in which the microbiome shapes our lives. The study of the human microbiome is not just a scientific endeavor; it is a journey into one of the most intimate and influential parts of our being, offering insights and opportunities to enhance our health and well-being in ways we are only just beginning to understand.

Understanding the Ecosystem in Your Gut

The human gut is more than just a digestive organ; it's a bustling metropolis of microorganisms, each playing a vital role in our overall health. This ecosystem, known as the gut microbiome, is a complex and dynamic environment, intricately connected to various aspects of our physical and mental well-being. This chapter aims to unravel the mysteries of this internal ecosystem, shedding light on how it functions, its critical importance, and how it interacts with the rest of the body.

The gut microbiome consists of trillions of microorganisms, including bacteria, viruses, fungi, and protozoa. These inhabitants are not random; they form a carefully balanced and interdependent community. The diversity of this microbial population is staggering, with hundreds of different species coexisting within the human gut. Each species has its unique role, from digesting food and synthesizing vitamins to training the immune system and communicating with the brain.

One of the most fascinating aspects of the gut microbiome is its symbiotic relationship with the human body. These microorganisms are not mere passengers; they are active participants in our health. In exchange for a habitat and nutrients, they perform a myriad of functions essential for our survival. For example, certain gut bacteria are responsible for breaking down dietary fiber into short-chain fatty acids, which are crucial for gut health and have anti-inflammatory effects.

The composition of the gut microbiome is influenced by various factors, including genetics, diet, lifestyle, and environmental exposures. Diet, in particular, plays a significant role in shaping the microbiome. Foods rich in fiber, such as fruits, vegetables, and whole grains, promote the growth of beneficial bacteria, while a diet high in processed foods can lead to a decrease in microbial diversity. This dynamic nature of the microbiome means that our dietary and lifestyle choices can have a profound impact on its composition and, consequently, our health.

The gut microbiome's role in immunity is another critical aspect of its functionality. It acts as a first line of defense against pathogens, preventing harmful bacteria from colonizing the gut. Additionally, it helps to educate and regulate the immune system, ensuring that it responds appropriately to potential threats. This interaction is crucial in preventing autoimmune diseases and allergies, where the immune system reacts inappropriately to harmless substances.

Beyond physical health, the gut microbiome is also intricately linked to mental health. The gut-brain axis, a two-way communication system between the gut and the brain, allows the microbiome to influence mood, stress levels, and even behavior. This connection is mediated by various mechanisms, including the production of neurotransmitters, immune signaling, and metabolic pathways. The implications of this relationship are far-reaching, offering new perspectives on treating conditions like depression, anxiety, and stress-related disorders.

The health of the gut microbiome is not just about preventing disease; it's about promoting overall well-being. A healthy and diverse microbiome is associated with numerous benefits, including improved digestion, enhanced immune function, and a reduced risk of chronic diseases like obesity, diabetes, and heart disease. Maintaining a healthy gut microbiome involves a combination of a balanced diet, regular exercise, stress management, and avoiding unnecessary antibiotics, which can disrupt the microbial balance.

Recent advances in science and technology have provided new tools for studying the gut microbiome, leading to groundbreaking discoveries and a deeper understanding of its complexities. These developments have opened the door to personalized medicine approaches, where treatments and dietary recommendations can be tailored to an individual's unique microbiome composition. This personalized approach has the potential to revolutionize health-care, making it more effective and customized to individual needs.

In conclusion, the ecosystem in our gut is a vital aspect of our health, influencing everything from digestion and immunity to mood and mental well-being. Understanding this complex and dynamic environment is key to maintaining good health and pre-venting disease. As we continue to explore and learn more about the gut microbiome, we are gaining valuable insights into how to care for this crucial part of our body. The gut microbiome is not just an internal ecosystem; it's a reflection of our lifestyle and choices, and nurturing it can lead to a healthier, happier life.

Key Players in Gut Health: Bacteria, Viruses, Fungi

The gut microbiome is a complex and dynamic community, teem-ing with a variety of microorganisms, each playing a crucial role in maintaining gut health. Among these, bacteria, viruses, and fungi stand out as key players, each contributing uniquely to the gut's ecosystem. This chapter aims to shed light on these diverse inhab-itants of the gut and explore their individual and collective roles in maintaining health and preventing disease.

Bacteria: The Frontline Workers of the Gut

Bacteria are the most studied and understood components of the gut microbiome. They are incredibly diverse, with hundreds of dif-ferent species cohabiting in the human gut. Each bacterial species has specific functions that contribute to the host's health. Some bacteria are adept at breaking down dietary fibers into short-chain fatty acids (SCFAs), such as butyrate, propionate, and acetate. These SCFAs are vital for gut health, serving as energy sources for gut cells and possessing anti-inflammatory properties.

Bacteria also play a pivotal role in synthesizing vitamins and other essential nutrients. For instance, some gut bacteria are responsible for producing vitamin K and certain B vitamins, crucial for blood clotting and energy metabolism. Moreover, the bacterial community in the gut helps in the development and functioning of the immune system, training immune cells to distinguish between harmful and benign entities.

Viruses: The Overlooked Influencers

Viruses in the gut, particularly bacteriophages (viruses that infect bacteria), are garnering increased attention for their role in shaping the gut microbiome. Bacteriophages can impact the composition of the bacterial community by infecting and lysing specific bacterial cells. This action not only controls bacterial populations but can also influence the overall diversity and stability of the microbiome.

Viruses contribute to horizontal gene transfer among bacteria, a process where genetic material is exchanged between bacterial cells. This transfer can lead to the emergence of beneficial traits, such as antibiotic resistance or the ability to metabolize certain dietary components. As such, viruses play a significant role in the adaptability and resilience of the gut microbiome.

Fungi: The Silent Partners

Fungi, though present in smaller numbers compared to bacteria, are an essential component of the gut microbiome. They include various yeast and mold species, each with specific roles in gut health. Fungi interact with bacteria and viruses, forming complex relationships that can influence the overall health of the gut ecosystem.

One of the critical functions of fungi in the gut is their involvement in the breakdown of complex carbohydrates, complementing the actions of bacteria. They also play a role in the immune system, with certain fungi known to stimulate immune responses. These interactions help maintain a balanced gut environment, preventing the overgrowth of harmful microorganisms and supporting the gut's barrier function.

Interactions and Balance: The Key to Gut Health

The health of the gut microbiome is not solely dependent on the presence of these microorganisms but on their interactions and balance. A diverse and balanced microbiome is associated with good health, while imbalances, known as dysbiosis, can lead to a range of health issues, including inflammatory bowel disease, obesity, and even mental health disorders.

Diet plays a crucial role in maintaining this balance. Foods rich in fiber, prebiotics, and probiotics can promote the growth of beneficial bacteria, viruses, and fungi, enhancing gut health. Conversely, a diet high in processed foods, sugars, and unhealthy fats can disrupt this balance, leading to dysbiosis.

Emerging research in microbiome science is continually revealing new insights into the roles of bacteria, viruses, and fungi in the gut. This research is not only deepening our understanding of gut health but also paving the way for new therapeutic strategies. Probiotics (live beneficial bacteria), prebiotics (compounds that feed beneficial bacteria), and even phage therapy (using bacteriophages to target specific bacteria) are being explored as potential treatments for various gut-related disorders.

In conclusion, bacteria, viruses, and fungi are key players in maintaining gut health. Their complex interactions and balance are crucial for the proper functioning of the gut and overall health. Understanding these microorganisms and their roles opens up new avenues for promoting gut health and preventing disease. As we continue to explore the depths of the gut microbiome, we are likely to uncover even more ways in which these microorganisms influence our health, offering new opportunities for targeted and effective treatments. The gut microbiome, with its diverse inhabitants, stands as a testament to the complexity and resilience of our internal ecosystems, highlighting the intricate connections between diet, microorganisms, and health.

Chapter 3: Foundations of Microbial Health

How the Microbiome Develops from Birth

The development of the human microbiome is a remarkable process that begins at birth and plays a crucial role in shaping our overall health. This intricate and dynamic process involves the gradual colonization of our bodies by a diverse array of microorganisms, primarily bacteria, which come to form the complex ecosystem known as the microbiome. Understanding how the microbiome develops from birth is essential in appreciating its impact on our health and well-being throughout life.

The Initial Colonization

At birth, a baby's sterile gut begins to be colonized by microorganisms. The mode of delivery has a significant impact on the initial composition of the microbiome. Babies born via vaginal delivery are exposed to their mother's vaginal and fecal microbes, which start the colonization process. In contrast, those born through cesarean section are more likely to be colonized by skin microbes and the hospital environment, leading to a different initial microbial composition.

Breastfeeding and Microbial Development

Breastfeeding plays a pivotal role in the development of the infant gut microbiome. Breast milk contains not only nutrients but also a variety of beneficial bacteria and bioactive compounds, including oligosaccharides, which act as prebiotics, stimulating the growth of beneficial gut bacteria. This composition helps in building a healthy and diverse microbiome, providing the infant with a robust start in life.

Dietary Influences

As infants transition to solid foods, their microbiome undergoes significant changes. The introduction of new foods diversifies the gut microbiota, introducing new species and strains. Diets rich in fruits, vegetables, and whole grains promote a diverse and healthy microbiome, while processed foods and sugars can lead to imbalances, affecting the child's health.

Environmental Exposures

The environment in which a child is raised also influences the development of their microbiome. Exposure to pets, siblings, and outdoor environments introduces a variety of microbes, contributing to microbial diversity. This exposure is thought to be beneficial, as it may help in developing a robust immune system and reducing the risk of allergies and autoimmune diseases.

Role of Antibiotics

Antibiotic use during early childhood can have a significant impact on the microbiome. Antibiotics can disrupt the delicate balance of the gut microbiota, leading to long-term changes in its composition. While sometimes necessary for treating infections, judicious use of antibiotics is crucial to prevent unnecessary disturbances in the developing microbiome.

The Maturing Microbiome

As children grow, their microbiome continues to evolve, becoming more stable and similar to the adult microbiome by late childhood. This maturation process is influenced by diet, lifestyle, and health status. A balanced and diverse microbiome is essential for proper digestion, immune function, and even mental health.

Microbiome and Immune System Development

The development of the microbiome is closely linked to the maturation of the immune system. A diverse microbiome trains the immune system to recognize and respond appropriately to various stimuli, including pathogens and harmless substances. This training is crucial in preventing overactive immune responses, such as allergies and autoimmune diseases.

Long-term Health Implications

The composition of the microbiome established during early life can have long-lasting effects on health. A healthy and balanced microbiome is associated with a lower risk of chronic diseases such as obesity, diabetes, and inflammatory bowel disease. In contrast, an imbalanced microbiome can predispose to these conditions, underscoring the importance of nurturing the microbiome from an early age.

The Future of Microbiome Research

Ongoing research is focused on understanding the intricate details of how the microbiome develops and its long-term health implications. This research holds promise for developing strategies to optimize microbiome health from birth, potentially preventing a range of diseases and promoting overall well-being.

In conclusion, the development of the microbiome from birth is a complex and dynamic process that plays a critical role in our health. The initial colonization, influenced by the mode of delivery and early diet, sets the stage for the microbial ecosystem that will inhabit our bodies throughout life. Environmental exposures, dietary choices, and the use of antibiotics further shape the developing microbiome. Understanding this process is key to appreciating the importance of the microbiome in health and disease, offering opportunities for early interventions to promote lifelong health. The microbiome's journey from birth is a testament to the intricate interplay between our bodies and the microbial world, highlighting the profound impact of this relationship on our health and well-being.

Factors Affecting Microbiome Composition

The composition of the human microbiome, particularly the gut microbiome, is a dynamic and complex entity, influenced by a myriad of factors throughout an individual's life. Understanding these factors is crucial in comprehending how changes in the microbiome can impact overall health. This chapter delves into the various elements that play a significant role in shaping the microbiome, highlighting their implications for health and disease.

Genetic Factors

Genetics play a foundational role in determining the initial landscape of an individual's microbiome. While the microbiome itself is not inherited in the traditional sense, genetic makeup can influence its composition. For example, genetic variations can affect the body's immune response, which in turn can shape the microbial community. However, it's important to note that while genetics provides a blueprint, it's the environmental and lifestyle factors that largely dictate the microbiome's diversity and abundance.

Birth Method

The process of birth is one of the first major events that influence the microbiome. Babies born vaginally are exposed to their mother's vaginal and gut microbiota, whereas those delivered via cesarean section are more likely to be colonized by skin microbes and the hospital environment. This initial exposure can have lasting effects on the infant's microbiome development and is linked to various health outcomes in later life.

Diet and Nutrition

Diet is one of the most significant and modifiable factors affecting the microbiome. The types of food consumed can dramatically alter the composition and function of the gut microbiota. Diets rich in fiber, such as those containing fruits, vegetables, and whole grains, support the growth of beneficial bacteria that produce short-chain fatty acids (SCFAs), crucial for gut health. Conversely, diets high in processed foods, sugar, and unhealthy fats can lead to a decrease in microbial diversity and an increase in harmful bacteria.

Lifestyle and Environment

Lifestyle choices and environmental exposures also play a crucial role. Factors such as physical activity, stress levels, and exposure to pollutants and chemicals can influence the microbiome. Regular exercise, for instance, has been shown to increase gut microbial diversity. High stress levels, on the other hand, can negatively impact the microbiome, potentially leading to dysbiosis.

Antibiotic Use

Antibiotics, while life-saving, can have a profound impact on the microbiome. They work by killing harmful bacteria causing infections but can also indiscriminately target beneficial gut bacteria. This can lead to a temporary reduction in microbial diversity and sometimes result in long-term changes to the microbiome, affecting overall health.

Age

The composition of the microbiome changes with age. In infancy and early childhood, the microbiome is quite variable and sensitive to external influences. As one ages, the microbiome tends to become more stable but can be altered by factors such as diet, lifestyle, and health status. In older age, the diversity of the microbiome often decreases, which has been linked to various age-related health issues.

Geographic and Cultural Influences

Geographical location and culture can influence the microbiome through diet, lifestyle, and environmental factors. For example, people living in rural areas often have a more diverse microbiome compared to those in urban areas, possibly due to different dietary habits and exposure to a wider range of environmental microbes.

Illness and Disease

Certain diseases and health conditions can also impact the microbiome. Conditions like inflammatory bowel disease, obesity, and type 2 diabetes have been linked to specific changes in the gut microbiota. The relationship can be bidirectional, where the disease affects the microbiome, and changes in the microbiome can influence the disease's progression.

Medications and Supplements

Apart from antibiotics, other medications and dietary supplements can affect the microbiome. For example, proton pump inhibitors, used to treat acid reflux, can alter gut bacteria, and certain dietary supplements, like probiotics, can introduce beneficial bacteria to the gut.

Psychological Factors

Emerging research suggests that psychological factors like stress and mood can also influence the microbiome. The gut-brain axis provides a pathway through which psychological states can impact gut health, demonstrating a complex interplay between mental health and the microbiome.

In conclusion, the composition of the human microbiome is shaped by a complex interplay of genetic, environmental, dietary, and lifestyle factors. This dynamic ecosystem is sensitive to changes and can significantly impact health and disease. Understanding these factors offers insights into maintaining a healthy microbiome and opens avenues for personalized approaches to health and medicine. By acknowledging and addressing these influences, we can better manage our microbiome, ultimately enhancing our overall health and well-being.

The Role of Genetics and Environment

In the intricate world of the human microbiome, two fundamental forces shape its composition and functionality: genetics and environment. These intertwined factors play a critical role in the development and maintenance of our microbial health, influencing everything from the diversity of our gut flora to our susceptibility to diseases. Understanding the interplay between genetics and environment is key to unraveling the complexities of the microbiome and its profound impact on our health.

Genetics: The Inherited Blueprint

Genetics provides the initial framework for the microbiome's development. Although we do not inherit the microbiome itself, our genetic makeup influences its composition. Genetic factors can dictate the environment of the gut, affecting its pH, immune responses, and the secretion of various substances that either foster or inhibit the growth of certain microbial species. For instance, variations in genes related to immune function can impact how our bodies interact with gut microbes, shaping the microbial community.

Additionally, genetics can influence the resilience and stability of the microbiome. Some individuals might have a genetic predisposition that allows their microbiome to bounce back quickly after disturbances like antibiotic use or illness. Others may experience more significant shifts in microbial composition due to the same factors, which could have lasting effects on their health.

Environment: Shaping the Microbial Landscape

While genetics lays the foundation, the environment plays a dynamic role in shaping the microbiome throughout life. Environmental factors encompass a broad range of elements, from the microbes we are exposed to at birth to the diet, lifestyle, and even the geographical location we inhabit.

Birth and Early Life

The initial colonization of the microbiome is profoundly influenced by the environment at birth. Vaginal births expose infants to a diverse range of microbes from the mother, which helps kickstart the development of a healthy microbiome. In contrast, cesarean births may lead to a different microbial composition, often influenced by skin and environmental bacteria.

Diet

Diet is perhaps the most significant environmental factor affecting the microbiome. Dietary patterns shape the gut's microbial population by providing substrates for bacterial growth. High-fiber diets, rich in fruits, vegetables, and whole grains, promote the growth of beneficial bacteria and the production of health-promoting short-chain fatty acids. Conversely, diets high in processed foods and sugars can lead to an overgrowth of pathogenic bacteria and reduce microbial diversity.

Lifestyle Factors

Lifestyle choices, including physical activity, smoking, and alcohol consumption, also impact the microbiome. Regular exercise, for instance, has been linked to increased gut microbial diversity. Smoking and excessive alcohol consumption, on the other hand, can have detrimental effects on the microbiome, contributing to dysbiosis and inflammation.

Environmental Exposures

Exposure to different environments, such as rural or urban settings, affects the microbiome by altering the range of microbial exposures. Urban environments, often characterized by higher pollution levels and reduced contact with natural environments, can lead to a less diverse microbiome compared to rural settings.

Antibiotic Use

Antibiotics significantly impact the microbiome by killing not only the targeted pathogens but also beneficial bacteria. This can lead to short-term disruptions and, in some cases, long-term changes in the microbiome's composition, underscoring the importance of cautious and judicious use of antibiotics.

The Interplay of Genetics and Environment

The relationship between genetics and environmental factors is complex and dynamic. While our genes provide a certain predisposition, it is the environmental exposures, particularly in early life, that play a crucial role in the actual development and composition of the microbiome. This interplay continues throughout life, with lifestyle choices and external factors continually influencing the microbiome's balance.

Understanding the combined influence of genetics and environment on the microbiome is vital for developing personalized approaches to health and disease management. It opens the door to targeted interventions that can modify the microbiome to promote health and prevent or treat diseases.

In conclusion, the development and maintenance of a healthy microbiome are profoundly influenced by both genetics and environmental factors. While our genetic makeup sets the stage, it is the environment that plays a leading role in shaping the microbial community within us. Recognizing the significance of these factors is key to unlocking the potential of microbiome research and its applications in health and medicine. As we continue to explore this fascinating interplay, we gain deeper insights into the intricate connections between our bodies, our environment, and the microscopic world that thrives within us.

Chapter 4: The Gut-Brain Connection

Unraveling the Gut-Brain Axis

The gut-brain axis, a complex communication network linking the gastrointestinal tract and the brain, stands at the frontier of modern medical research. This bi-directional pathway not only reflects the physical connection between the gut and the brain but also embodies the intricate interplay between our mental health and gastrointestinal function. Understanding the gut-brain axis is crucial in comprehending how gut health can impact brain function and vice versa, offering new insights into the treatment of both gastrointestinal and neurological disorders.

The Biological Basis of the Gut-Brain Axis

The gut-brain axis primarily operates through neural, hormonal, and immune pathways, facilitating constant communication between the gut microbiota and the brain. The enteric nervous system, often referred to as the "second brain," contains millions of neurons that govern gastrointestinal function and directly communicate with the brain via the vagus nerve. This neural pathway allows for rapid signaling between the gut and the brain, influencing mood, cognitive functions, and gut motility.

Hormonal signals also play a critical role. The gut produces a variety of hormones and neurotransmitters, some of which are identical to those found in the brain, such as serotonin and gamma-aminobutyric acid (GABA). These substances can affect mood and behavior, illustrating how changes in the gut microbiome can directly impact mental health.

The immune system is another vital link in the gut-brain axis. The gut microbiota influences immune responses, and in turn, the immune system modulates gut-brain communication. Inflammation in the gut can lead to inflammatory responses in the brain, contributing to neurological conditions like depression and anxiety.

Impact on Mental Health

Recent studies have shed light on the gut-brain axis's role in mental health. For example, alterations in gut microbiota have been associated with mood disorders such as depression and anxiety. The mechanism behind this involves the production of neurotransmitters by gut bacteria, the modulation of inflammation, and the impact of gut hormones on brain function. This connection opens up new avenues for treating mental health disorders by targeting the gut microbiome with probiotics, dietary changes, and lifestyle modifications.

Influence on Gastrointestinal Disorders

The gut-brain axis also has implications for gastrointestinal health. Stress and anxiety can exacerbate symptoms of gastrointestinal disorders like irritable bowel syndrome (IBS) and inflammatory bowel disease (IBD). This occurs through the stress-induced activation of the hypothalamic-pituitary-adrenal (HPA) axis, leading to changes in gut motility, barrier function, and microbiota composition. Understanding this connection can lead to more effective treatments that address both the psychological and physiological aspects of these disorders.

The Role of Diet and Nutrition

Diet is a critical modulator of the gut-brain axis. Foods rich in probiotics and prebiotics can positively influence gut health, which in turn can have beneficial effects on mental health. Dietary interventions that enhance microbial diversity in the gut can lead to improved mood, cognition, and reduction in stress-related symptoms.

Stress and the Gut-Brain Connection

Chronic stress is a major disruptor of the gut-brain axis. It can lead to alterations in gut microbiota, increased intestinal permeability (leaky gut), and changes in gut motility. These changes can exacerbate gastrointestinal symptoms and have been linked to the development of certain mental health disorders.

Future Directions in Research and Treatment

The exploration of the gut-brain axis is leading to novel therapeutic strategies for a range of conditions. For example, the use of psychobiotics, beneficial bacteria with the potential to improve mental health, is an area of growing interest. Furthermore, understanding the gut-brain connection is enhancing our approach to treating gastrointestinal disorders, incorporating stress management, and psychological therapies alongside traditional treatments.

Personalized Medicine and the Gut-Brain Axis

The gut-brain axis also has significant implications for personalized medicine. Since each individual's microbiome is unique, treatments targeting the gut-brain axis can be tailored to individual needs, offering more effective and personalized care.

In conclusion, the gut-brain axis is a complex and dynamic interface integral to our understanding of health and disease. It underscores the interdependence of mental and gastrointestinal health, challenging the traditional view of these as separate entities. As research in this area continues to evolve, it holds the promise of revolutionizing the treatment of both mental health and gastrointestinal disorders, highlighting the importance of holistic approaches in medicine. The gut-brain axis is not just a pathway of communication; it is a symbol of the intricate and profound connections that govern our bodies and our health.

Microbiome's Influence on Mood and Mental Health

In recent years, the burgeoning field of psychobiotics has brought to light the profound influence of the gut microbiome on mood and mental health. The intricate network known as the gut-brain axis, which connects the gut microbiome with the brain, has been identified as a key player in this interaction. This chapter delves into how the microbiome affects our psychological well-being, offering a new perspective on treating mental health disorders.

Understanding the Gut-Brain Connection

The gut-brain axis is a bi-directional communication system involving neural, hormonal, and immune pathways. This complex network allows the gut microbiota to send and receive signals to and from the brain. The enteric nervous system, often called the second brain, contains more neurons than the spinal cord and uses many of the same neurotransmitters as the brain, such as serotonin and GABA. These neurotransmitters play crucial roles in regulating mood and are significantly influenced by the state of the gut microbiome.

The Role of Microbial Metabolites

Microbial metabolites, such as short-chain fatty acids (SCFAs), produced during the fermentation of dietary fibers, have a significant impact on brain function. SCFAs can modulate the blood-brain barrier, influence immune response, and affect neuronal signaling, all of which play roles in mental health. The production of these metabolites depends largely on the composition of the gut microbiota, linking diet directly to mental well-being.

Neurotransmitter Production

Certain gut bacteria are capable of producing neurotransmitters that are key to mental health. For instance, some species are involved in synthesizing serotonin, a neurotransmitter that contributes to feelings of happiness and well-being. An imbalance in the gut microbiota can lead to altered levels of these neurotransmitters, potentially contributing to mood disorders.

Inflammation and Mental Health

Chronic inflammation, often a result of gut dysbiosis, is increasingly recognized as a contributing factor to various mental health conditions, including depression and anxiety. Pro-inflammatory cytokines produced in response to an imbalanced microbiome can impact the brain and alter mood and behavior. Reducing inflammation through modulation of the gut microbiota therefore offers a potential pathway for treating or even preventing certain mental health disorders.

Stress Response and the HPA Axis

The hypothalamic-pituitary-adrenal (HPA) axis, the body's central stress response system, is also influenced by the gut microbiome. An imbalanced microbiome can lead to an overactive HPA axis, resulting in heightened stress responses. This has implications for conditions like anxiety and depression, where stress response regulation is often disrupted.

The Potential of Psychobiotics

Psychobiotics, probiotics that have a beneficial impact on mental health, are an emerging area of interest. These beneficial bacteria can positively influence the gut-brain axis, potentially improving mood and cognitive function. While research in this field is still in its infancy, early studies suggest that certain probiotics could be useful adjuncts to traditional mental health treatments.

Dietary Influences on the Microbiome and Mental Health

Diet plays a crucial role in shaping the gut microbiome, and consequently, mental health. Diets rich in diverse plant-based foods support a healthy microbiome, promoting the production of beneficial metabolites and neurotransmitters. Conversely, diets high in processed foods can lead to an imbalanced microbiome, potentially impacting mental health.

Implications for Mental Health Treatment

Understanding the link between the microbiome and mental health opens up new avenues for treating psychiatric disorders. Integrating dietary and lifestyle modifications along with traditional psychiatric treatments could provide a more holistic approach to mental health care. This could include personalized dietary recommendations to support a healthy microbiome, alongside psychological therapies and medications.

Future Directions in Research

As research in this area continues to grow, the potential for new, innovative treatments for mental health disorders expands. Future studies are likely to provide deeper insights into the specific mechanisms by which the microbiome influences mental health and how these can be targeted therapeutically.

In conclusion, the influence of the gut microbiome on mood and mental health is a groundbreaking discovery in the field of mental health research. The gut-brain axis offers a complex yet fascinating window into the interplay between our gut health and psychological well-being. As we continue to unravel the mysteries of this connection, the potential for new, more effective treatments for mental health disorders becomes increasingly apparent. This new understanding also underscores the importance of holistic approaches to health, considering both the physical and mental aspects of well-being. The exploration of the microbiome's influence on mental health is not just a scientific journey; it's a pathway to a deeper understanding of the human condition and the intricate connections that govern our health and happiness.

Case Studies: Anxiety, Depression, and Beyond

The burgeoning research into the gut-brain axis has begun to illuminate the profound impact of the gut microbiome on mental health conditions like anxiety and depression. Through various case studies, scientists and clinicians are unraveling the intricate ways in which the microbiome influences these disorders, providing insights that could revolutionize their treatment. This chapter delves into several key case studies that highlight the relationship between the gut microbiome and mental health disorders, offering a glimpse into the future of mental health treatment.

Anxiety and the Microbiome

In one landmark study, researchers explored the impact of the gut microbiome on anxiety-like behaviors in mice. They observed that mice raised in a germ-free environment exhibited higher levels of anxiety compared to their normal counterparts. Remarkably, when these germ-free mice were colonized with a healthy microbiome, their anxiety levels decreased, suggesting a direct link between gut health and anxiety.

Further human studies have corroborated these findings. For instance, a clinical trial examined the effects of probiotics on individuals with anxiety. Participants who consumed a probiotic-rich diet for several weeks reported significant reductions in anxiety symptoms. These changes were also accompanied by alterations in brain regions associated with emotional processing, as observed through functional MRI scans.

Depression and Gut Dysbiosis

Depression has also been linked to changes in the gut microbiome. Researchers have found distinct differences in the composition of the gut microbiota in individuals with depression compared to healthy controls. These differences include decreased levels of certain beneficial bacteria known to produce neuroactive substances like serotonin and dopamine.

In a pivotal study, fecal microbiota transplantation (FMT) from depressed patients to germ-free mice resulted in the mice exhibiting depressive-like behaviors. This remarkable finding provided compelling evidence for the role of the gut microbiome in modulating mood and behavior.

Beyond Anxiety and Depression

The influence of the gut microbiome extends beyond anxiety and depression to other mental health conditions. For example, research has begun to explore the microbiome's role in disorders such as autism spectrum disorder (ASD), schizophrenia, and bipolar disorder.

In the case of ASD, several studies have reported alterations in the gut microbiome composition of affected individuals. Some research suggests that these microbial changes may be linked to certain symptoms of ASD, such as gastrointestinal issues and behavioral problems. While the exact mechanisms remain unclear, these findings point to the gut microbiome as a potential target for therapeutic intervention.

Therapeutic Implications

These case studies have significant implications for the treatment of mental health disorders. The use of probiotics, prebiotics, and even FMT are being explored as potential treatments. The idea of "feeding the gut" to heal the mind is gaining traction, with dietary interventions becoming an integral part of holistic mental health treatment plans.

Challenges and Future Directions

Despite these promising findings, there are challenges in translating them into effective treatments. The complexity of the gut-brain axis and individual variations in microbiome composition mean that a one-size-fits-all approach is unlikely to be effective. Future research will need to focus on personalized treatments based on individual microbiome profiles.

Additionally, more extensive and rigorous clinical trials are required to fully understand the therapeutic potential and limitations of manipulating the gut microbiome in treating mental health disorders. This includes deciphering the complex interactions between diet, microbiome composition, and mental health.

The Holistic Approach to Mental Health

These case studies underscore the importance of a holistic approach to mental health. They highlight the need to consider not just the brain but also the gut in understanding and treating mental health disorders. This paradigm shift could lead to more effective and comprehensive treatment strategies that address both psychological and physiological factors.

In conclusion, the case studies examining the relationship between the gut microbiome and mental health disorders like anxiety, depression, and beyond are paving the way for a new understanding of mental health. They reveal a complex but potentially modifiable factor in these conditions – the gut microbiome. As research in this field continues to grow, it holds the promise of more targeted and effective treatments, offering hope to millions of people affected by mental health disorders. This research not only challenges our traditional views of mental health but also opens up a world of new possibilities for treatment and prevention, solidifying the importance of the gut-brain connection in our overall well-being.

Chapter 5: Gut Microbiome and Physical Health

The Microbiome's Impact on Digestive Wellness

The gut microbiome, a complex and dynamic community of microorganisms residing in our gastrointestinal tract, plays a pivotal role in digestive wellness. This community, predominantly composed of bacteria but also including viruses, fungi, and protozoa, is essential for various aspects of digestion and gut health. The growing body of research on the gut microbiome has shed light on its crucial role in maintaining digestive wellness, offering new perspectives on the treatment and prevention of various digestive disorders.

Digestion and Nutrient Absorption

One of the primary roles of the gut microbiome is aiding in the digestion of food and the absorption of nutrients. The microbiome facilitates the breakdown of complex carbohydrates, fibers, and certain proteins and fats that the human body cannot digest on its own. This process not only allows us to extract more energy and nutrients from our food but also results in the production of beneficial compounds like short-chain fatty acids (SCFAs). SCFAs, including butyrate, propionate, and acetate, are crucial for maintaining the health and integrity of the gut lining, offering protection against diseases like colorectal cancer.

Gut Barrier and Immune Function

The gut microbiome plays a critical role in maintaining the gut barrier and modulating immune function. A healthy microbiome strengthens the gut barrier, preventing harmful substances and pathogens from entering the bloodstream. This function is crucial in preventing inflammation and infections. Moreover, the microbiome interacts with the gut-associated lymphoid tissue (GALT), a key component of the immune system, helping to train immune cells and regulate immune responses. This interaction is vital in preventing overactive immune responses and autoimmune conditions.

Gut Microbiome and Gastrointestinal Disorders

An imbalance in the gut microbiome, known as dysbiosis, has been linked to various gastrointestinal disorders, including irritable bowel syndrome (IBS), inflammatory bowel disease (IBD), and gastroesophageal reflux disease (GERD). In cases of IBS and IBD, dysbiosis can lead to increased gut permeability (leaky gut), inflammation, and altered gut motility, contributing to the symptoms of these disorders. Research into the microbiome's role in these conditions is offering new insights into their pathogenesis and potential treatment strategies, including the use of probiotics, prebiotics, and dietary interventions.

The Role in Metabolic Health

The gut microbiome also has significant implications for metabolic health. It influences the metabolism of bile acids, cholesterol, and other lipids, impacting the risk of conditions like obesity and type 2 diabetes. Certain gut bacteria can affect insulin sensitivity and the metabolic response to dietary components, further linking gut health to overall metabolic wellness.

The Microbiome and Gut-Brain Axis

The gut-brain axis, a communication network linking the gut microbiome with the brain, has implications for digestive wellness. Stress and emotional states can influence gut motility, secretion, and inflammation, which in turn can impact gut health. Conversely, a healthy gut microbiome can positively affect mood and stress responses, illustrating the bidirectional nature of this relationship.

Diet and the Microbiome

Diet is a major modulator of the gut microbiome. Diets rich in diverse, plant-based foods support a healthy and diverse microbiome, promoting good digestion and reducing the risk of gastrointestinal disorders. On the other hand, diets high in processed foods, sugars, and unhealthy fats can lead to dysbiosis, contributing to poor digestive health.

Future Directions in Gut Health Research

Research into the gut microbiome is continually evolving, offering new insights into its role in digestive wellness. This research is not only enhancing our understanding of gut health but also paving the way for novel therapeutic approaches, such as personalized microbiome-based treatments. The field of fecal microbiota transplantation (FMT) is particularly promising in treating conditions like Clostridioides difficile infection and is being explored for other gastrointestinal disorders.

The Holistic Approach to Digestive Health

Understanding the microbiome's impact on digestive wellness underscores the need for a holistic approach to gut health. This approach includes not only medical treatments but also dietary and lifestyle interventions to support a healthy microbiome. Such strategies can improve digestive function, prevent gastrointestinal disorders, and enhance overall health and well-being.

In conclusion, the gut microbiome's role in digestive wellness is multifaceted and profound. It plays a crucial role in digestion, nutrient absorption, immune function, and the prevention of gastrointestinal disorders. As we continue to uncover the complexities of the gut microbiome, its significance in digestive health becomes increasingly apparent, offering new opportunities for maintaining and improving gut health. The exploration of the microbiome's impact on digestive wellness is not just a scientific endeavor; it's a journey towards a deeper understanding of how we can harness the power of these microscopic inhabitants for better health and quality of life.

Microbial Influence on Immune Function

The human gut microbiome, a diverse community of microorganisms residing in the gastrointestinal tract, is a crucial player in the regulation and maintenance of the immune system. The interaction between gut microbes and the immune system is a complex, bidirectional relationship that is vital for both the prevention of disease and the maintenance of overall health. This chapter explores how the gut microbiome influences immune function, shedding light on the interconnectedness of our microbial inhabitants and our body's defense mechanisms.

The Gut Microbiome as an Immune Modulator

The gut microbiome is intricately involved in the development and education of the immune system. From early life, exposure to a diverse range of microbes in the gut helps train the immune system to distinguish between harmful pathogens and harmless substances, including food particles and beneficial bacteria. This training is essential for developing a balanced immune response, preventing overreactions that can lead to allergies and autoimmune diseases.

Barrier Function and Pathogen Defense

One of the primary roles of the gut microbiome in immune function is the maintenance of the intestinal barrier. A healthy microbiome strengthens the gut lining, preventing the leakage of harmful substances and pathogens into the bloodstream. This barrier function is crucial in protecting the body from infections and inflammation. Certain gut bacteria produce substances like short-chain fatty acids, which reinforce the barrier integrity and regulate immune cell function.

Microbial Metabolites and Immune Signaling

Microbial metabolites, such as SCFAs, play significant roles in immune signaling. These metabolites can influence the behavior of immune cells both within the gut and throughout the body. For example, butyrate, a SCFA produced by bacterial fermentation of dietary fibers, has anti-inflammatory properties and can modulate the activity of T cells, a type of white blood cell critical for immune response.

Immune Tolerance and Autoimmunity

The gut microbiome is instrumental in developing immune tolerance, the process by which the immune system learns to be unresponsive to harmless substances. Imbalances in the gut microbiota, or dysbiosis, can disrupt this tolerance, potentially leading to autoimmune conditions where the body mistakenly attacks its own tissues. Studies have linked certain autoimmune diseases, like type 1 diabetes and rheumatoid arthritis, to alterations in the gut microbiome.

The Role in Inflammation and Chronic Disease

Chronic inflammation, a root cause of many diseases, is closely linked to the state of the gut microbiome. An imbalanced microbiome can trigger an inappropriate immune response, leading to systemic inflammation. This inflammation is a contributing factor in a wide range of conditions, including heart disease, obesity, and metabolic syndrome.

The Impact of Diet and Lifestyle

Diet and lifestyle have profound impacts on the composition of the gut microbiome and, consequently, on immune function. Diets rich in fiber, fruits, and vegetables promote the growth of beneficial microbes that support immune health. Conversely, diets high in processed foods and sugars can lead to dysbiosis and impaired immune responses. Lifestyle factors such as stress, sleep, and exercise also influence the microbiome and immune health.

Probiotics and Immune Health

Probiotics, beneficial bacteria found in certain foods and supplements, can positively influence immune function. These bacteria can restore balance to the gut microbiome, enhance barrier function, and modulate immune responses. Probiotics have shown promise in reducing the incidence and severity of respiratory infections, gastrointestinal infections, and even some autoimmune diseases.

Future Directions in Research and Therapeutics

Research into the gut microbiome's role in immune function is rapidly advancing, offering new insights into the prevention and treatment of diseases. The development of microbiome-based therapies, such as personalized probiotics and fecal microbiota transplantation, is an area of growing interest. These therapies hold the potential to treat a range of conditions by restoring microbial balance and promoting healthy immune responses.

Conclusion

The influence of the gut microbiome on immune function is a testament to the complex interplay between our body and its microbial inhabitants. A healthy, balanced gut microbiome is critical for robust immune function, protecting against pathogens, regulating inflammation, and preventing autoimmune diseases. As our understanding of this intricate relationship grows, so does the potential for innovative treatments that harness the power of the microbiome to enhance immune health. The gut microbiome's role in immune function is not just a fascinating area of research; it is a crucial aspect of our health and well-being, highlighting the importance of maintaining a healthy microbial ecosystem for optimal immune function.

Link Between the Microbiome and Chronic Diseases

The gut microbiome, a complex ecosystem of microorganisms residing in our gastrointestinal tract, has emerged as a significant factor in the development and progression of various chronic diseases. This intricate microbial community exerts a profound influence on our overall health, extending far beyond the digestive system. In recent years, research has increasingly focused on how imbalances in the gut microbiome, known as dysbiosis, are linked to the onset and exacerbation of chronic diseases such as obesity, diabetes, cardiovascular diseases, and certain types of cancer.

The Microbiome and Obesity

Obesity, a growing global health concern, has been closely linked to the state of the gut microbiome. Studies have shown that individuals with obesity often have a less diverse gut microbiome compared to those of a healthy weight. This reduced diversity can affect metabolic functions, including energy extraction from food and fat storage. Certain bacteria in the gut are more efficient at extracting calories from food, and their overrepresentation can contribute to weight gain. Furthermore, dysbiosis can lead to inflammation, which is a known risk factor for obesity and related metabolic disorders.

Diabetes and Microbial Imbalances

Type 2 diabetes, characterized by insulin resistance and high blood sugar levels, has also been associated with changes in the gut microbiome. Research indicates that individuals with type 2 diabetes often have different gut microbial compositions compared to healthy individuals. These changes can impair the gut's ability to produce and regulate certain hormones that affect insulin sensitivity and glucose metabolism. Additionally, some gut bacteria can influence inflammation, a key factor in the development of insulin resistance.

Cardiovascular Health and the Microbiome

The gut microbiome's role in cardiovascular health is an area of intense study. Certain gut bacteria are involved in the metabolism of dietary components like choline and L-carnitine, leading to the production of trimethylamine N-oxide (TMAO), a compound associated with an increased risk of heart disease. Moreover, dysbiosis can contribute to chronic inflammation, a significant risk factor for atherosclerosis, hypertension, and stroke.

The Gut Microbiome and Cancer

Emerging research suggests a link between the gut microbiome and certain types of cancer, particularly colorectal cancer. The gut microbiome can influence the gut's health and integrity, and certain bacterial species have been associated with increased inflammation and DNA damage, which can lead to cancer. Some bacteria also produce carcinogenic compounds that can contribute to the development of colorectal cancer.

Inflammatory Bowel Disease (IBD)

IBD, including Crohn's disease and ulcerative colitis, is a chronic inflammatory condition of the gastrointestinal tract. While the exact cause of IBD is unknown, it is clear that dysbiosis plays a crucial role. Patients with IBD often exhibit significant alterations in their gut microbiota, with a decrease in anti-inflammatory bacteria and an increase in pro-inflammatory bacteria. This imbalance contributes to the chronic inflammation characteristic of IBD.

The Role of Diet and Lifestyle

Diet and lifestyle significantly impact the composition and health of the gut microbiome, thereby influencing the risk of chronic diseases. Diets high in fiber and low in processed foods promote a healthy and diverse microbiome, which can mitigate the risk of chronic diseases. Conversely, diets high in processed foods, sugars, and unhealthy fats can lead to dysbiosis and an increased risk of these conditions. Lifestyle factors such as physical activity, stress management, and sleep also play roles in maintaining a healthy microbiome.

Therapeutic Implications

Understanding the link between the microbiome and chronic diseases has significant implications for prevention and treatment. Modulating the gut microbiome through diet, probiotics, prebiotics, and even fecal microbiota transplantation offers potential avenues for managing and treating chronic diseases. These strategies aim to restore a healthy balance in the gut microbiome, thereby reducing inflammation and other risk factors associated with chronic diseases.

Future Directions in Microbiome Research

Research into the microbiome's role in chronic diseases is rapidly advancing, with the potential to significantly alter our approach to these conditions. Future studies are likely to focus on identifying specific microbial patterns associated with different chronic diseases and developing targeted interventions to modulate the microbiome effectively.

In conclusion, the link between the gut microbiome and chronic diseases is a critical area of modern medical research. The gut microbiome's influence extends far beyond the digestive system, impacting our risk and experience of various chronic diseases. As our understanding of this complex microbial ecosystem grows, so does the potential for innovative treatments and preventive measures. The gut microbiome's role in chronic diseases underscores the importance of maintaining a healthy and balanced microbial community, highlighting the interconnectedness of our lifestyle choices, our microbiome, and our long-term health.

Chapter 6: Diet and Your Microbiome

How Food Choices Shape Your Gut Health

The adage "you are what you eat" holds profound truth when it comes to the gut microbiome. Our dietary habits play a pivotal role in shaping the composition and functionality of the trillions of microorganisms residing in our gastrointestinal tract. This chapter explores how different food choices can significantly influence gut health, affecting everything from digestive processes to immune function and even mental well-being.

The Impact of Diet on Microbial Diversity

Diversity in the gut microbiome is a key indicator of good health. A varied and balanced diet rich in whole foods provides a wide range of nutrients that foster a diverse microbial community. Each type of food can promote the growth of specific bacterial populations. For instance, high-fiber foods such as fruits, vegetables, and whole grains are fermented by gut bacteria into beneficial short-chain fatty acids (SCFAs), which are crucial for gut health.

The Role of Fiber

Dietary fiber plays a starring role in gut health. It acts as a prebiotic, providing food for beneficial gut bacteria. These bacteria ferment fiber, producing SCFAs like butyrate, which nourish gut cells, reduce inflammation, and strengthen the gut barrier. Diets low in fiber, conversely, can lead to reduced microbial diversity and lower SCFA production, potentially increasing the risk of gut-related disorders.

Probiotics and Fermented Foods

Fermented foods like yogurt, kefir, sauerkraut, and kimchi are rich in probiotics, beneficial bacteria that can augment the gut microbiome. Consuming these foods can introduce new beneficial bacteria to the gut, enhancing its diversity and functionality. Probiotics have been shown to be beneficial in managing conditions like irritable bowel syndrome (IBS) and promoting overall gut health.

The Effects of Processed Foods

In contrast to whole foods, highly processed foods can have detrimental effects on gut health. These foods often contain additives, preservatives, and high levels of sugar and unhealthy fats, which can promote the growth of harmful bacteria and yeast. This shift in the microbial balance can lead to dysbiosis, a state of imbalance in the microbiome, associated with various health issues, including obesity, diabetes, and inflammatory bowel disease.

Impact of Sugar on the Microbiome

High sugar intake can significantly impact the gut microbiome. Sugars can feed certain harmful bacteria and yeast, like Candida, leading to overgrowth and imbalances. This can disrupt the gut barrier, increase inflammation, and impair immune function. Reducing sugar intake is thus crucial for maintaining a healthy and balanced microbiome.

Role of Plant-Based Diets

Plant-based diets, rich in fruits, vegetables, legumes, nuts, and seeds, are particularly beneficial for gut health. They provide a wide range of fibers, antioxidants, and phytonutrients that promote a diverse and healthy microbiome. These diets have been linked to lower risks of gut inflammation, colorectal cancer, and other digestive disorders.

Animal Proteins and Gut Health

Animal proteins, when consumed in moderation, can be part of a healthy diet. However, excessive consumption of red and processed meats has been associated with negative changes in the gut microbiome. These foods can lead to the proliferation of bacteria that produce harmful substances like TMAO, linked to cardiovascular disease. Balancing animal proteins with plenty of plant-based foods is key for a healthy microbiome.

The Importance of Fats

The type of fats in our diet also influences the gut microbiome. Omega-3 fatty acids, found in fish, flaxseeds, and walnuts, have anti-inflammatory effects and can positively impact gut health. In contrast, saturated and trans fats, often found in processed foods, can promote inflammation and negatively affect the microbiome.

Personalized Nutrition for Gut Health

Emerging research suggests that the impact of diet on the gut microbiome may vary from person to person. This has led to a growing interest in personalized nutrition, where dietary recommendations are tailored to an individual's unique microbiome composition. Such approaches hold promise for optimizing gut health based on personal dietary responses.

Conclusion

Our food choices have a profound impact on the health and composition of our gut microbiome. A diet rich in diverse, whole foods supports a healthy and balanced microbial community, crucial for overall health. Conversely, diets high in processed foods, sugars, and unhealthy fats can lead to microbial imbalances and a range of health issues. Understanding the relationship between diet and gut health is key to making informed food choices that nurture our microbiome and enhance our well-being. As research in this field continues to evolve, the role of diet in shaping our gut microbiome remains a fundamental aspect of health and disease prevention.

Superfoods for Your Microbiome

In the realm of gut health, the term "superfoods" refers to foods that are particularly beneficial for the gut microbiome. These foods are rich in nutrients that promote the growth of beneficial bacteria, enhance gut barrier function, and contribute to overall digestive wellness. Incorporating these superfoods into your diet can lead to a healthier, more balanced gut microbiome, which is essential for overall health. This chapter explores a variety of superfoods and their benefits for the gut microbiome.

The Power of Fiber-Rich Foods

Fiber is a cornerstone nutrient for the gut microbiome, and foods rich in dietary fiber are considered superfoods for gut health. These include fruits, vegetables, whole grains, legumes, nuts, and seeds. The fiber in these foods is not digested by human enzymes but is fermented by gut bacteria, producing short-chain fatty acids (SC-FAs) like butyrate, which are essential for maintaining the health of gut cells and reducing inflammation.

Fruits and Vegetables

Fruits and vegetables are packed with fiber, vitamins, minerals, and antioxidants. Dark leafy greens, such as spinach and kale, are particularly beneficial as they are high in fiber and nutrients. Berries, apples, and bananas are also excellent choices, providing prebiotic fiber that feeds beneficial gut bacteria.

Whole Grains

Whole grains like oats, barley, and quinoa are excellent sources of complex carbohydrates and fiber. They support a diverse and healthy microbiome by providing the necessary substrate for beneficial bacterial fermentation.

Legumes

Beans, lentils, and chickpeas are high in fiber and protein, making them superb foods for gut health. They contain resistant starch, which passes through the small intestine undigested and is fermented in the colon, promoting the growth of beneficial bacteria.

Fermented Foods: Probiotic Powerhouses

Fermented foods are natural sources of probiotics, beneficial bacteria that can help balance the gut microbiome. Including these foods in your diet can introduce new beneficial strains of bacteria to the gut.

Yogurt and Kefir

Yogurt and kefir are rich in probiotics and can help replenish and diversify the gut microbiota. They also contain calcium and protein, contributing to overall health.

Sauerkraut and Kimchi

Fermented vegetables like sauerkraut and kimchi are not only probiotic-rich but also contain vitamins and fiber. The fermentation process enhances the bioavailability of nutrients and introduces beneficial bacteria.

Miso and Tempeh

Miso, a fermented soybean paste, and tempeh, a fermented soybean product, are traditional components of Asian cuisine. They are excellent sources of probiotics and plant-based protein.

Prebiotic Foods

Prebiotics are dietary fibers that the human body cannot digest but are fermented by gut bacteria. They help stimulate the growth of beneficial bacteria in the gut.

Garlic and Onions

Garlic and onions are rich in inulin and fructooligosaccharides, two effective prebiotics. They promote the growth of beneficial Bifidobacteria and Lactobacilli in the gut.

Asparagus and Leeks

Asparagus and leeks are other excellent sources of prebiotic fibers. They support a healthy gut microbiome by providing the fuel that beneficial gut bacteria need to thrive.

Polyphenol-Rich Foods

Polyphenols are plant compounds with antioxidant properties. They are not always fully absorbed in the small intestine and thus make their way to the colon, where they are metabolized by gut bacteria.

Dark Chocolate and Berries

Dark chocolate and berries, especially blueberries, are rich in polyphenols. These compounds can promote the growth of beneficial bacteria and inhibit the growth of harmful bacteria.

Green Tea

Green tea is another excellent source of polyphenols. Regular consumption of green tea has been associated with an increase in beneficial bacteria like Bifidobacteria.

Omega-3 Fatty Acids

Omega-3 fatty acids, found in fatty fish, flaxseeds, and walnuts, are known for their anti-inflammatory properties. They can help reduce gut inflammation and are beneficial for overall gut health.

Fatty Fish

Fatty fish like salmon, mackerel, and sardines are high in omega-3 fatty acids and are excellent for gut health. They help modulate the gut microbiome and reduce inflammation.

Conclusion

Incorporating a variety of superfoods into your diet can significantly benefit your gut microbiome. These foods provide the necessary nutrients to promote the growth of beneficial bacteria, enhance gut barrier function, and reduce inflammation. By focusing on a diet rich in fiber, probiotics, prebiotics, polyphenols, and omega-3 fatty acids, you can support your gut health and, by extension, your overall health and well-being. A healthy gut microbiome is not just about preventing digestive disorders; it's a key component of a holistic approach

Balancing Your Diet for Optimal Microbial Diversity

In the intricate ecosystem of the human gut, microbial diversity is a hallmark of health and resilience. The vast array of microorganisms that reside within our gastrointestinal tract thrives on a varied diet, rich in different nutrients and compounds. Understanding how to balance your diet to promote this diversity is essential for optimal gut health and, by extension, overall well-being. This chapter explores the principles of a balanced diet that nurtures microbial diversity, providing practical insights into fostering a healthy gut microbiome.

The Foundation of a Microbiome-Friendly Diet

A diet that promotes microbial diversity is rich in a variety of plant-based foods. These foods provide a range of fibers, prebiotics, and phytonutrients that feed different types of beneficial bacteria in the gut. Incorporating a wide array of fruits, vegetables, whole grains, legumes, nuts, and seeds ensures that your microbiome receives a diverse spectrum of nutrients necessary for its health.

The Role of Fiber in Microbial Diversity

Dietary fiber is perhaps the most crucial component for a diverse microbiome. Found in plant-based foods, fiber is not digested by human enzymes but is fermented by gut bacteria. This fermentation process not only produces beneficial short-chain fatty acids (SCFAs) like butyrate but also fosters a varied bacterial population. Each type of fiber feeds different bacterial species, so eating a wide range of fibrous foods is key.

Incorporating a Rainbow of Fruits and Vegetables

Fruits and vegetables are not only rich in fiber but also contain various phytonutrients, vitamins, and minerals that benefit the microbiome. Each color in fruits and vegetables represents different nutrients and antioxidants. For instance, the red in tomatoes and strawberries comes from lycopene, while the purple in blueberries and eggplants is a sign of anthocyanins. These compounds can have prebiotic effects and support a healthy gut environment.

The Importance of Whole Grains

Whole grains like oats, barley, quinoa, and brown rice are excellent sources of complex carbohydrates, fibers, and B vitamins. Unlike refined grains, whole grains retain their nutrient-rich bran and germ, providing a feast for gut bacteria. They help in maintaining a balanced microbiome and contribute to overall digestive health.

The Benefits of Legumes

Legumes, including beans, lentils, and chickpeas, are not only excellent sources of plant-based protein but also rich in fibers and resistant starch. These components are key for feeding beneficial gut bacteria and promoting SCFA production, crucial for gut health.

Nuts and Seeds: Microbiome Superchargers

Nuts and seeds are packed with fibers, healthy fats, and a variety of vitamins and minerals. They add diversity to the diet and are beneficial for the gut microbiome. Almonds, for instance, are high in prebiotic fibers that can increase beneficial bacterial populations.

Balancing Animal Proteins

While a plant-centric diet is beneficial for the microbiome, animal proteins can also be part of a balanced diet. It's important to choose lean and high-quality sources like poultry, fish, eggs, and dairy. Fatty fish, in particular, are rich in omega-3 fatty acids, which have anti-inflammatory properties beneficial for gut health. Moderation and variety are key in incorporating animal proteins into a microbiome-friendly diet.

Limiting Processed Foods and Sugars

Processed foods and high-sugar diets can negatively impact microbial diversity. These foods can promote the growth of harmful bacteria and yeast, leading to dysbiosis, a microbial imbalance. Reducing the intake of processed foods, artificial additives, and sugars is crucial for maintaining a healthy and diverse gut microbiome.

Hydration and Gut Health

Adequate hydration is essential for digestive health and, consequently, for a healthy microbiome. Water aids in digestion and helps maintain the mucosal lining of the intestines, providing a healthy environment for gut bacteria.

Personalizing Your Diet

Each person's microbiome is unique, so the response to different foods can vary. Listening to your body and observing how it responds to certain foods is important. Some people may find they digest certain foods better than others, and this can be a guide to personalizing their diet for optimal gut health.

Conclusion

Balancing your diet for optimal microbial diversity is about incorporating a wide range of nutrient-rich foods, focusing on plant-based ingredients, and limiting processed foods and sugars. This dietary approach not only supports a diverse and healthy gut microbiome but also contributes to overall health and disease prevention. Understanding the impact of your dietary choices on your gut microbiome is a powerful tool for maintaining wellness and vitality. As research continues to uncover the complex relationships between diet, the microbiome, and health, the importance of a balanced, diverse diet becomes ever more clear.

Chapter 7: Lifestyle and Microbial Health

Stress, Sleep, and the Microbiome

The intricate relationship between our lifestyle factors, such as stress and sleep, and the gut microbiome is a rapidly evolving area of scientific inquiry. The gut microbiome, which plays a crucial role in our overall health, is not only affected by what we eat but also by how we live. Both stress and sleep have profound impacts on the composition and function of our gut microbiome, influencing everything from digestion to mental health. This chapter delves into the complex interactions between stress, sleep, and the microbiome, offering insights into how these lifestyle factors can either support or hinder microbial health.

The Impact of Stress on the Gut Microbiome

Stress, whether acute or chronic, can significantly alter the gut microbiome. The body's stress response triggers the release of various hormones, including cortisol, which can affect gut motility, secretion, and permeability. These physiological changes can create an environment in the gut that favors the growth of certain bacteria over others, potentially leading to dysbiosis, an imbalance in the microbial community.

Stress-Induced Dysbiosis

Stress-induced dysbiosis can have several consequences for health. For example, it can impair the integrity of the gut barrier, leading to increased gut permeability, commonly known as leaky gut. This condition allows bacteria and toxins to "leak" into the bloodstream, triggering inflammation and immune responses. Chronic inflammation, in turn, has been linked to various health issues, including mental health disorders, obesity, and autoimmune diseases.

Stress Management and Microbial Health

Managing stress is thus crucial for maintaining a healthy gut microbiome. Practices such as mindfulness meditation, yoga, and regular exercise have been shown to mitigate the impact of stress on the gut microbiome. These activities reduce stress hormone levels and promote a more balanced gut environment, supporting microbial diversity and function.

The Role of Sleep in Microbial Health

Sleep, much like diet and stress, plays a significant role in the health of the gut microbiome. Adequate, high-quality sleep is essential for the proper functioning of the immune system, hormone regulation, and cognitive processes, all of which are interconnected with gut health.

Sleep Disruption and the Microbiome

Disruptions in sleep patterns, such as those caused by shift work, jet lag, or sleep disorders, can lead to changes in the gut microbiome. Altered sleep can disturb the circadian rhythms of gut microbes, impacting their metabolic activity and potentially leading to dysbiosis. This dysbiosis can contribute to metabolic disturbances, such as insulin resistance and weight gain, and negatively affect mental health.

Promoting Healthy Sleep

To support a healthy gut microbiome, prioritizing good sleep hygiene is essential. This includes maintaining a regular sleep schedule, creating a restful sleeping environment, and avoiding stimulants like caffeine and electronic devices before bedtime. Good sleep practices not only benefit the gut microbiome but also enhance overall health and well-being.

The Bidirectional Relationship Between the Microbiome, Stress, and Sleep

The relationship between stress, sleep, and the gut microbiome is bidirectional. Just as stress and poor sleep can negatively impact the microbiome, an imbalanced microbiome can exacerbate stress responses and disrupt sleep patterns. For instance, gut dysbiosis can lead to the production of inflammatory cytokines, which can affect mood and stress levels. Similarly, changes in the gut microbiome can influence the production of neurotransmitters like serotonin, much of which is produced in the gut and is crucial for regulating sleep.

Integrating Diet, Stress Management, and Sleep

To optimize gut health, it is important to integrate dietary choices with stress management and sleep hygiene. A balanced diet rich in fiber, probiotics, and prebiotics supports a healthy microbiome, which can mitigate the negative effects of stress and improve sleep quality. Conversely, managing stress and ensuring adequate sleep can enhance the gut's ability to respond to a healthy diet, creating a positive feedback loop that supports overall health.

Conclusion

The interplay between stress, sleep, and the gut microbiome highlights the importance of a holistic approach to health. By acknowledging the impact of these lifestyle factors on our microbial inhabitants, we can adopt practices that promote microbial balance and diversity. Managing stress, prioritizing sleep, and making mindful dietary choices are key strategies for maintaining a healthy gut microbiome. As research continues to unravel the complexities of the gut-brain axis, the connections between our lifestyle, our microbiome, and our health become increasingly clear, underscoring the significance of our daily choices in shaping our overall well-being.

Exercise and Gut Health

In recent years, the link between physical activity and gut health has garnered significant attention in the field of health and wellness. Exercise, known for its myriad benefits to the cardiovascular system, muscles, and mental health, also plays a crucial role in shaping the gut microbiome. This chapter delves into the multifaceted relationship between exercise and gut health, exploring how physical activity influences the diversity and functionality of our gut microbiota.

The Influence of Exercise on Microbial Diversity

Regular physical activity is associated with increased diversity in the gut microbiome. A diverse microbiome is generally considered a marker of good gut health, as it indicates a wide range of functional capabilities and resilience against pathogenic invasions. Studies have shown that athletes and physically active individuals tend to have a more diverse gut microbiota compared to sedentary individuals. This diversity is linked to enhanced metabolic health, improved immune function, and reduced inflammation.

Mechanisms Behind Exercise-Induced Microbial Changes

The mechanisms by which exercise promotes a healthy and diverse microbiome are multifaceted. Physical activity can alter the gut environment in ways that favor the growth of beneficial bacteria. Exercise-induced changes in the body's metabolism can lead to alterations in the production of bile acids, fatty acids, and other substances that can influence microbial growth. Additionally, the physical act of moving the body can stimulate bowel movements, improving gut motility and the overall health of the gastrointestinal tract.

Exercise and Short-Chain Fatty Acids (SCFAs)

One significant benefit of exercise on gut health is its impact on the production of short-chain fatty acids (SCFAs), such as butyrate, propionate, and acetate. These compounds, produced by the fermentation of dietary fibers by gut bacteria, play critical roles in maintaining gut barrier integrity, modulating immune responses, and providing energy for gut cells. Regular exercise can enhance the production of SCFAs, leading to a healthier gut lining and reduced risk of inflammatory diseases.

Exercise, Gut Inflammation, and Immune Function

Regular physical activity can also influence gut inflammation and immune function. Exercise has been shown to reduce inflammation in the gut, which can be beneficial for individuals with inflammatory bowel diseases (IBD) like Crohn's disease and ulcerative colitis. The anti-inflammatory effects of exercise are partly due to changes in the gut microbiome and increased production of SCFAs. Furthermore, exercise can enhance the body's immune responses, partly through its effects on the gut-associated lymphoid tissue (GALT), a key component of the immune system in the gut.

The Role of Exercise in Gut-Brain Axis

The gut-brain axis, a communication network linking the gut microbiome with the brain, is also influenced by exercise. Physical activity can improve mood and reduce stress, partly through its positive effects on the gut microbiome. A healthy gut microbiome can produce neurotransmitters and other bioactive molecules that influence brain function, suggesting a pathway through which exercise can benefit mental health.

Balancing Exercise Intensity for Optimal Gut Health

While moderate exercise is beneficial for gut health, it's important to note that excessive or intense physical activity can sometimes have adverse effects on the gut. High-intensity exercise, especially without adequate rest and recovery, can lead to gastrointestinal disturbances and increased intestinal permeability, commonly known as "leaky gut." Therefore, balancing exercise intensity and ensuring proper recovery is crucial for reaping the gut health benefits of physical activity.

Exercise, Diet, and the Microbiome

The benefits of exercise on the gut microbiome can be further enhanced when combined with a healthy diet. A diet rich in fibers, prebiotics, and probiotics supports the growth of beneficial gut bacteria and maximizes the positive effects of exercise on the microbiome. Consuming a balanced diet that includes a variety of plant-based foods can synergize with regular physical activity to promote a healthy and diverse gut microbiome.

Conclusion

Exercise is a powerful modulator of gut health, capable of enhancing microbial diversity, reducing inflammation, and improving overall gut function. Its role in promoting a healthy gut microbiome adds another layer to the already extensive benefits of regular physical activity. By incorporating moderate, balanced exercise into our daily routines, we can support our gut health and, by extension, our overall well-being. As research continues to unfold the complex interactions between physical activity and the gut microbiome, the message is clear: moving our bodies is not just about building muscles or cardiovascular health; it's also about nurturing the billions of microorganisms that reside within us and play a crucial role in our health.

Environmental Factors Influencing Microbial Balance

The environment in which we live plays a significant role in shaping our gut microbiome, affecting everything from its composition to its functionality. Environmental factors, ranging from the air we breathe to the water we drink, and even the soil where our food grows, can influence the delicate balance of our gut microbiota. This chapter explores various environmental factors and their impacts on microbial balance, offering insights into how our surroundings are intrinsically linked to our gut health.

Exposure to Microbes in Early Life

The development of the gut microbiome begins at birth and is heavily influenced by the initial environmental exposures. Infants delivered vaginally are exposed to their mother's vaginal microbiota, while those born via cesarean section are more likely to be colonized by skin microbes and those present in the hospital environment. This early exposure plays a crucial role in seeding the infant's gut microbiome.

Breastfeeding further shapes the infant's gut microbiome, as breast milk contains a variety of beneficial bacteria and oligosaccharides that act as prebiotics. In contrast, formula-fed infants often have different microbial compositions. These early life exposures set the stage for the gut microbiome's future development.

The Role of Diet and Food Sources

The diet is one of the most influential environmental factors affecting the gut microbiome. Foods that are rich in fiber, such as fruits, vegetables, and whole grains, promote the growth of beneficial bacteria. On the other hand, a diet high in processed foods, sugars, and unhealthy fats can lead to an imbalance in the microbiome, known as dysbiosis.

The source and quality of food also matter. Organically grown foods, which are less likely to contain pesticide residues, can have different impacts on the gut microbiome compared to conventionally grown produce. Similarly, the use of antibiotics in animal farming can affect the microbiome of meat consumers, potentially leading to antibiotic resistance and altered gut flora.

Urbanization and Its Effects

Urbanization and modern lifestyle changes have significant impacts on the gut microbiome. Urban environments tend to have less microbial diversity compared to rural environments. Limited exposure to diverse natural environments in urban settings can lead to a less diverse gut microbiome. This phenomenon is often referred to as the "hygiene hypothesis," suggesting that overly sterile environments can impede the proper development of the immune system and microbiome.

Pollution and Chemical Exposures

Exposure to environmental pollutants and chemicals can also influence the gut microbiome. Air pollution, heavy metals, and chemicals like bisphenol A (BPA) found in plastics can disrupt the balance of gut bacteria, leading to inflammation and increased risk of diseases. These pollutants can alter the gut environment, making it more hospitable for pathogenic bacteria and less so for beneficial ones.

Antibiotic Use and Microbial Balance

The widespread use of antibiotics, not just in healthcare but also in agriculture, has a profound impact on the gut microbiome. Antibiotics can indiscriminately kill both harmful and beneficial bacteria, leading to decreased microbial diversity and resilience. The overuse of antibiotics has been linked to increased risks of gut dysbiosis, obesity, and even mental health disorders.

Water Quality and Microbiome Health

The quality of water we consume is another environmental factor that can affect the gut microbiome. Water contaminated with pathogens, heavy metals, or industrial pollutants can disrupt the gut flora and lead to gastrointestinal diseases. Conversely, clean and safe drinking water supports the maintenance of a healthy gut microbiome.

The Importance of Green Spaces

Access to green spaces and natural environments has been shown to have a positive impact on the gut microbiome. Interacting with nature and its diverse microbial life can enhance the diversity of our gut microbiota. Regular exposure to natural environments, such as parks, forests, and gardens, is associated with improved gut health and overall well-being.

Conclusion

The relationship between environmental factors and the gut microbiome is complex and multifaceted. From the air we breathe to the food we eat and the water we drink, every aspect of our environment can have a significant impact on our gut health. Recognizing and understanding these influences is crucial in maintaining a balanced and healthy microbiome. As we become increasingly aware of these environmental impacts, it becomes essential to consider how our lifestyle choices and the spaces we inhabit contribute to our microbial well-being. By fostering environments that support microbial diversity and reduce exposure to harmful pollutants and chemicals, we can take proactive steps towards nurturing our gut microbiome and enhancing our overall health.

Chapter 8: Rebalancing Your Microbiome

Signs of Microbiome Imbalance

The gut microbiome, a complex and dynamic community of microorganisms in our gastrointestinal tract, plays a crucial role in our overall health. When this microbiome is in balance, it supports various bodily functions, from digestion to immune response. However, when imbalanced – a condition known as dysbiosis – it can lead to a range of health issues. Recognizing the signs of microbiome imbalance is key to addressing gut health issues and maintaining overall wellness. This chapter focuses on the common indicators of an imbalanced gut microbiome and the health implications associated with it.

Gastrointestinal Symptoms

One of the most direct signs of microbiome imbalance is a change in gastrointestinal symptoms. These can include:

Altered Bowel Movements

Changes in bowel habits, such as constipation, diarrhea, or a combination of both, can indicate dysbiosis. An imbalanced microbiome can disrupt normal gut motility, leading to these issues.

Bloating and Gas

Excessive bloating and gas are common signs of microbiome imbalance. Certain bacteria in the gut produce more gas than others, and an overgrowth of these bacteria can lead to discomfort and bloating.

Abdominal Pain

Persistent or recurrent abdominal pain can be a sign of an imbalanced gut microbiome. This pain can be a result of gas buildup, inflammation, or other gut disturbances caused by microbial dysbiosis.

Systemic Symptoms

The effects of a microbiome imbalance can extend beyond the gut, affecting the body systemically:

Fatigue

Chronic fatigue or a general feeling of low energy can be linked to gut health. The gut microbiome is involved in nutrient absorption and energy production, and an imbalance can lead to decreased efficiency in these processes.

Skin Conditions

The skin, often referred to as the 'mirror of the gut', can reflect an imbalanced microbiome. Conditions like eczema, acne, and psoriasis can be exacerbated by gut dysbiosis due to the inflammatory response it can trigger.

Food Sensitivities

An increase in food sensitivities or intolerances can be a sign of an imbalanced gut. Dysbiosis can lead to a weakened gut barrier, allowing food particles to enter the bloodstream and trigger immune responses.

Mental Health Impacts

The gut-brain axis, the communication pathway between the gut and the brain, means that gut health can significantly impact mental health:

Mood Fluctuations

Mood disorders, including anxiety and depression, have been linked to gut health. Dysbiosis can affect the production of neurotransmitters like serotonin, much of which is produced in the gut.

Cognitive Issues

Difficulties with concentration, memory, and overall cognitive function can sometimes be traced back to gut health. The inflammatory response associated with dysbiosis can have a detrimental effect on brain function.

Immune System Dysfunction

The gut microbiome plays a crucial role in immune system regulation:

Frequent Infections

If you find yourself catching infections more frequently, it could be a sign of a weakened immune system due to a compromised gut microbiome.

Autoimmune Conditions

Emerging research suggests a link between microbiome imbalance and the development of autoimmune diseases. The loss of microbial diversity can lead to an overactive immune response against the body's own tissues.

Weight Changes

Unexpected weight changes, either gain or loss, without significant changes in diet or exercise habits, can be a sign of microbiome imbalance:

Unexplained Weight Gain

An imbalanced microbiome can affect the body's metabolism and the way it processes food, sometimes leading to weight gain.

Difficulty Losing Weight

Similarly, an unhealthy gut microbiome can make it difficult to lose weight, even with a healthy diet and regular exercise.

How to Address Microbiome Imbalance

Recognizing these signs is the first step in addressing microbiome imbalance. The next steps involve dietary changes, lifestyle modifications, and possibly medical interventions:

Dietary Adjustments

Incorporating a diverse range of fiber-rich foods, probiotics, and prebiotics can help restore balance to the gut microbiome.

Lifestyle Changes

Reducing stress, getting adequate sleep, and regular physical activity can positively impact gut health.

Medical Consultation

If symptoms persist, it is important to consult a healthcare professional. They can provide guidance on appropriate treatments, which may include probiotics, prebiotic supplements, or in some cases, antibiotics or other medications.

Conclusion

Understanding the signs of microbiome imbalance is crucial in maintaining not just gut health, but overall health and well-being. By paying attention to these signs and taking proactive steps to address them, it is possible to restore balance to the gut microbiome. A balanced microbiome not only supports digestive health but also plays a significant role in immune function, mental health, and general vitality. As research continues to unfold the complexities of the gut microbiome, it becomes increasingly clear how critical it is to maintain this delicate balance for optimal health.

Probiotics, Prebiotics, and Synbiotics

In the quest to maintain or restore a healthy gut microbiome, probiotics, prebiotics, and synbiotics have emerged as key players. These dietary components work in different but complementary ways to promote a balanced and diverse gut microbiota, which is essential for overall health. This chapter delves into the nature of probiotics, prebiotics, and synbiotics, their roles in gut health, and how they can be integrated into everyday diet and lifestyle to support the microbiome.

Understanding Probiotics

Probiotics are live microorganisms, typically bacteria or yeast, which when consumed in adequate amounts, confer health benefits to the host. They are often referred to as 'good' or 'friendly' bacteria because they help balance the gut microbiome.

Sources of Probiotics

Probiotics are naturally found in fermented foods like yogurt, kefir, sauerkraut, kimchi, miso, and tempeh. They are also available as dietary supplements in various forms, including capsules, tablets, and powders.

Health Benefits

Probiotics can help restore the natural balance of gut bacteria, especially after it has been disrupted by illness, antibiotic treatment, or poor diet. They have been shown to be beneficial in managing gastrointestinal conditions like irritable bowel syndrome (IBS), inflammatory bowel diseases (IBD), and infectious diarrhea. Additionally, probiotics can enhance immune function, improve skin health, and may even have positive effects on mental health due to the gut-brain connection.

The Role of Prebiotics

Prebiotics are non-digestible food components that promote the growth of beneficial bacteria in the gut. Essentially, they act as food for probiotics and are crucial for maintaining a healthy gut microbiome.

Sources of Prebiotics

Prebiotics are found in many high-fiber foods, including fruits, vegetables, and whole grains. Specific examples include bananas, onions, garlic, leeks, asparagus, artichokes, and whole wheat. Prebiotics are also available as dietary supplements.

Health Implications

By feeding and stimulating the growth of beneficial bacteria, prebiotics help improve gut health. They have been linked to increased production of short-chain fatty acids (SCFAs), reduced risk of gastrointestinal disorders, better immune function, improved digestion, and enhanced nutrient absorption. Prebiotics can also play a role in regulating blood sugar levels and possibly in weight management.

Synbiotics: Combining Probiotics and Prebiotics

Synbiotics refer to nutritional supplements or foods that combine probiotics and prebiotics in a form of synergy. The idea behind synbiotics is that the prebiotic component will selectively stimulate the growth and activity of the probiotic component, thereby enhancing its benefits.

Composition and Benefits

A typical synbiotic product might contain a combination of a specific probiotic strain and a prebiotic fiber that is known to support the growth of that strain. The health benefits of synbiotics include all those associated with probiotics and prebiotics, with the potential for these effects to be more pronounced due to the synergistic interaction.

Integrating Probiotics, Prebiotics, and Synbiotics into Your Diet

Dietary Approach

The most natural way to incorporate probiotics and prebiotics into your diet is through food. Eating a diverse range of fermented foods can provide a variety of probiotic strains, while a high-fiber diet rich in fruits, vegetables, and whole grains will supply ample prebiotics.

Supplementation

For those looking to address specific health concerns or who are unable to get enough probiotics and prebiotics from their diet, supplements can be an effective option. It's important to choose high-quality supplements and, if possible, seek advice from a healthcare professional, especially when targeting specific health issues.

Considerations and Precautions

While probiotics and prebiotics are generally considered safe for most people, there are some considerations and precautions to keep in mind:

Individual Responses

The impact of probiotics and prebiotics can vary from person to person. Some individuals may experience gas and bloating, especially when first introducing these components into their diet.

Specific Health Conditions

People with certain health conditions, such as compromised immune systems, should consult healthcare professionals before taking probiotic or prebiotic supplements, as there may be risks involved.

Quality and Strain Specificity

Not all probiotic supplements are created equal, and different strains offer different benefits. It's crucial to choose supplements that are backed by science and contain viable strains.

Conclusion

Probiotics, prebiotics, and synbiotics represent important tools in the maintenance and restoration of a healthy gut microbiome. By understanding their roles and how to effectively incorporate them into your diet, you can take proactive steps towards improving your gut health. As research continues to unveil the complexities of the gut microbiome and its impact on overall health, the use of

probiotics, prebiotics, and synbiotics is likely to play an increasingly significant role in healthcare and wellness strategies. Their integration into daily life marks a shift towards a more holistic approach to health, emphasizing the importance of the gut in maintaining overall well-being.

A Guide to Resetting Your Gut Health

Resetting gut health is a journey that involves nurturing and rebalancing the delicate ecosystem of microorganisms residing in our gastrointestinal tract. Given the gut microbiome's profound impact on overall health, resetting it can lead to improved digestion, better immune function, enhanced mental health, and overall well-being. This chapter offers a comprehensive guide to resetting your gut health, focusing on diet, lifestyle changes, and other strategies to cultivate a healthy gut microbiome.

Understanding the Importance of Gut Health

The first step in resetting your gut health is understanding its significance. The gut microbiome plays a crucial role in digesting food, synthesizing nutrients, regulating the immune system, and even influencing mood and behavior. An imbalance in the gut microbiome, known as dysbiosis, can contribute to a range of health issues, including digestive disorders, obesity, autoimmune diseases, and mental health conditions.

Dietary Changes for a Healthy Microbiome

Increase Fiber Intake

Dietary fiber, found in fruits, vegetables, whole grains, legumes, nuts, and seeds, is essential for a healthy gut. Fiber serves as food for beneficial gut bacteria and aids in the production of short-chain fatty acids, which are vital for gut health.

Incorporate Fermented Foods

Fermented foods like yogurt, kefir, sauerkraut, kimchi, and kombucha are rich in probiotics. Including these in your diet can introduce beneficial bacteria to your gut.

Diversify Your Diet

Eating a wide variety of foods can promote a diverse microbiome, which is associated with better health. Try to include different colors of fruits and vegetables, various whole grains, and multiple protein sources.

Limit Processed Foods and Sugars

Processed foods and high-sugar diets can lead to an overgrowth of harmful bacteria. Reducing the intake of these foods is crucial in maintaining a balanced gut microbiome.

Lifestyle Modifications

Manage Stress

Chronic stress can negatively impact gut health. Engaging in stress-reduction techniques like meditation, yoga, deep breathing exercises, or regular physical activity can help maintain a healthy gut.

Prioritize Sleep

Adequate and quality sleep is essential for gut health. Establishing a regular sleep schedule and creating a restful environment can support the gut-brain axis and improve microbiome health.

Regular Exercise

Moderate exercise has been shown to increase gut microbial diversity and improve gut health. Incorporating regular physical activity into your routine can have lasting benefits for your gut microbiome.

Understanding Probiotics and Prebiotics

Probiotics

Probiotics are live microorganisms that provide health benefits when consumed. Supplementing with probiotics or consuming probiotic-rich foods can help restore gut bacterial balance.

Prebiotics

Prebiotics are non-digestible fibers that feed beneficial gut bacteria. Including prebiotic-rich foods like garlic, onions, leeks, asparagus, and bananas in your diet can support the growth of healthy gut bacteria.

Hydration

Maintaining adequate hydration is key to gut health. Water aids in digestion, nutrient absorption, and the elimination of waste, supporting overall gut function.

Elimination Diets and Food Sensitivities

If certain foods seem to trigger digestive discomfort, consider an elimination diet to identify and remove potential irritants. This process involves removing common triggers like gluten, dairy, soy, or certain FODMAPs and then gradually reintroducing them to pinpoint sensitivities.

Detoxifying the Body

While the concept of detoxification is often overstated, supporting your body's natural detoxification processes can benefit gut health. This involves limiting alcohol, avoiding environmental toxins, and

eating detoxifying foods like leafy greens and cruciferous vegetables.

Regular Medical Check-Ups

Regular check-ups with a healthcare professional can help monitor
gut health and address any issues. They can also offer guidance on
the use of probiotics, prebiotics, and other supplements.

Monitoring and Adjusting

Gut health is dynamic, so it's important to monitor how your body
responds to different foods and lifestyle changes. Keeping a food
and symptom diary can be a useful tool in understanding your
body's reactions and adjusting your approach accordingly.

Conclusion

Resetting your gut health is a multifaceted process that involves
making informed dietary choices, adopting beneficial lifestyle
habits, and understanding the role of probiotics and prebiotics.
By nurturing your gut microbiome, you can support your overall health and well-being. This guide provides the foundational
steps to embark on a journey towards a healthier, more balanced
gut. Remember, changes in the gut microbiome don't happen
overnight, and a consistent, mindful approach is key to achieving
lasting gut health.

Chapter 9: Innovations in Microbiome Research

Cutting-edge Research and Discoveries

The field of microbiome research is one of the most dynamic and rapidly evolving areas in modern science. Groundbreaking discoveries and technological advancements are continuously reshaping our understanding of the human microbiome and its profound impact on health and disease. This chapter delves into the latest research and discoveries in microbiome science, highlighting how these innovations are paving the way for new diagnostic tools, therapeutic strategies, and a deeper understanding of human biology.

Deciphering the Microbiome's Complexity

Recent advancements in genomic sequencing technologies have revolutionized our ability to analyze the microbiome. High-throughput sequencing techniques, such as 16S rRNA sequencing and whole-genome shotgun sequencing, have provided unprecedented insights into the complexity and diversity of microbial communities. Researchers are now able to identify and catalog the vast array of microorganisms that inhabit the human body, many of which were previously unknown.

Microbial Genomics and Metagenomics

The use of metagenomics, studying genetic material recovered directly from environmental samples, has been particularly transformative. This approach allows scientists to study the collective genome of the microbiome, providing a comprehensive picture of its composition, functionality, and interactions with the host.

The Gut-Brain Axis: Unraveling the Connection

One of the most exciting areas of microbiome research is the exploration of the gut-brain axis. Scientists are uncovering how the gut microbiome influences brain health and behavior, offering new perspectives on neurological and psychiatric disorders.

Microbiome and Mental Health

Studies are increasingly showing links between gut microbial composition and conditions such as depression, anxiety, and autism spectrum disorder. Researchers are exploring how microbial byproducts, immune signaling, and neural pathways connect the gut and brain, opening the door to potential microbiome-based treatments for mental health issues.

Personalized Microbiome Therapies

The concept of personalized medicine is being extended to microbiome research. Recognizing that each individual's microbiome is unique, scientists are developing personalized approaches to treating diseases through microbiome modulation.

Fecal Microbiota Transplantation (FMT)

FMT, the process of transferring fecal bacteria from a healthy donor to a patient, is being studied for its effectiveness in treating various conditions, including Clostridioides difficile infection, IBD, and even obesity. The potential of FMT lies in its ability to quickly restore microbial balance in the gut.

Designer Probiotics

Another promising area is the development of designer probiotics – genetically engineered bacteria designed to perform specific functions in the gut, such as producing therapeutic compounds or targeting pathogenic bacteria.

The Microbiome and Chronic Diseases

Research is increasingly focusing on the role of the microbiome in chronic diseases such as obesity, diabetes, cardiovascular disease, and certain types of cancer. Studies are exploring how dysbiosis contributes to the pathogenesis of these conditions and how restoring microbial balance can be a part of treatment and prevention strategies.

Microbiome as a Diagnostic Tool

The potential of the microbiome as a diagnostic tool is also being explored. Specific microbial signatures are being linked to certain diseases, suggesting that analyzing an individual's microbiome could aid in early detection and personalized treatment plans.

Impact of Diet and Lifestyle

The interplay between diet, lifestyle, and the microbiome is a key area of research. Scientists are examining how different foods, dietary patterns, and lifestyle factors such as exercise and stress management affect the microbiome. This research is crucial for developing dietary guidelines and lifestyle interventions that support microbiome health.

Environmental Influences

Researchers are also investigating how environmental factors, including exposure to antibiotics, pollutants, and toxins, impact the microbiome. This line of inquiry is critical for understanding how modern living conditions are affecting our microbiome and what changes might be necessary to protect it.

Future Directions and Challenges

As microbiome research continues to advance, several challenges and future directions emerge:

Ethical and Privacy Concerns

With the increase in microbiome data collection, ethical and privacy issues related to genetic information are becoming more prominent. Addressing these concerns is crucial for the continued advancement of the field.

Integrative Approaches

Future research will likely take a more holistic approach, integrating microbiome studies with other areas such as genomics, metabolomics, and immunology, to gain a more comprehensive understanding of human health.

Global Microbiome Initiatives

There is a growing recognition of the need for large-scale, global studies of the microbiome. Such initiatives can provide valuable insights into how different lifestyles, diets, and environments affect the microbiome across diverse populations.

Conclusion

The cutting-edge research and discoveries in microbiome science are fundamentally changing our understanding of human health. From unraveling the complexities of the gut-brain axis to developing personalized microbiome therapies, these advancements are at the forefront of a new era in medicine and healthcare. As we continue to explore the intricate world of the human microbiome, the potential for innovative treatments, improved diagnostics, and enhanced understanding of human biology grows ever more promising.

Personalized Microbiome Analysis

In the ever-evolving landscape of health and wellness, personalized microbiome analysis stands out as a groundbreaking innovation. This cutting-edge approach involves examining an individual's unique microbiome composition to provide tailored health recommendations. Such analysis marks a significant shift from the one-size-fits-all approach to a more individualized strategy in healthcare. This chapter explores the concept, techniques, and implications of personalized microbiome analysis and how it is reshaping our approach to health and disease.

The Concept of Personalized Microbiome Analysis

Personalized microbiome analysis is based on the premise that each individual's gut microbiome is unique. Factors like genetics, diet, lifestyle, and environmental exposures contribute to this uniqueness. By analyzing an individual's microbiome, scientists and healthcare providers can gain insights into their specific health risks, dietary needs, and even predispositions to certain diseases.

Techniques in Microbiome Analysis

Advancements in genomic sequencing technologies have made personalized microbiome analysis possible. Techniques such as 16S rRNA sequencing and whole-genome shotgun sequencing allow for detailed identification and quantification of the microorganisms present in an individual's gut.

16S rRNA Sequencing

This method targets a specific region of the microbial genetic material, which is highly conserved among different species, allowing for the identification and classification of bacteria.

Whole-Genome Shotgun Sequencing

This more comprehensive technique sequences all the genetic material in a microbiome sample, providing a detailed overview of the microbial community, including bacteria, viruses, fungi, and protozoa.

Applications in Health and Disease

Personalized microbiome analysis has numerous applications in understanding and managing health and disease. By assessing an individual's microbiome, it's possible to identify imbalances or dysbiosis, which can be linked to various health issues.

Digestive Health

Personalized microbiome analysis can reveal specific bacterial populations linked to conditions like IBS, IBD, and celiac disease, aiding in targeted treatment approaches.

Weight Management

The analysis can provide insights into the microbiome's role in metabolism and obesity, helping tailor dietary recommendations for weight management.

Chronic Disease Risk

Studies have linked certain microbial patterns to the risk of chronic diseases like diabetes, heart disease, and certain cancers. Personalized analysis can help in early detection and preventive strategies.

Mental Health

Given the gut-brain axis connection, microbiome analysis can also offer information relevant to mental health conditions like depression and anxiety.

Personalized Dietary Recommendations

One of the most exciting applications of personalized microbiome analysis is in the field of nutrition. By understanding the specific needs and responses of an individual's microbiome, dietary recommendations can be tailored for optimal health.

Prebiotics and Probiotics

Analysis can guide the selection of specific prebiotic fibers and probiotic strains that would be most beneficial for an individual's gut health.

Food Sensitivities

Identifying how certain foods affect the microbiome can help in pinpointing food sensitivities or intolerances, allowing for more personalized diet plans.

Challenges and Considerations

While the potential of personalized microbiome analysis is vast, there are several challenges and considerations in its application.

Interpretation and Actionability

Interpreting the complex data from microbiome analysis and translating it into actionable health advice requires expertise and a deep understanding of microbiome science.

Privacy and Ethical Concerns

Handling sensitive genetic information responsibly is crucial. There are privacy and ethical considerations regarding the collection, storage, and use of such personal data.

Cost and Accessibility

Currently, the cost of comprehensive microbiome analysis can be prohibitive for many, and access to these technologies is not universally available.

Future Directions

The field of personalized microbiome analysis is rapidly evolving, with ongoing research expanding its potential applications.

Integrative Health Approaches

Future developments may see more integrative approaches, combining microbiome analysis with other health data for a holistic view of an individual's health.

Predictive Modeling

Advancements in bioinformatics may lead to predictive models that can anticipate how changes in the microbiome could affect health, allowing for proactive health management.

Broader Accessibility

As technology advances and costs decrease, personalized microbiome analysis may become more accessible, making it a standard part of health assessments.

Conclusion

Personalized microbiome analysis represents a significant leap forward in our ability to understand and manage health at an individual level. By tailoring health recommendations based on the unique composition of one's microbiome, we can move closer to more effective, personalized healthcare. This approach not only has the potential to improve outcomes for individuals but also offers a broader understanding of the human microbiome and its critical role in health and disease. As we continue to explore and understand the complex interactions within our microbiome, the possibilities for enhanced health and wellness through personalized analysis and interventions become increasingly promising.

Future Therapies and Treatments

The exploration of the human microbiome has opened new frontiers in medical science, particularly in the development of innovative therapies and treatments. As we continue to unravel the complexities of the microbiome, its profound impact on human health is becoming increasingly evident. This chapter focuses on the potential future therapies and treatments emerging from microbiome research, promising a revolution in healthcare and a shift towards more personalized and effective medical interventions.

Microbiome-based Therapeutics

The realization that the gut microbiome plays a critical role in health and disease has led to the exploration of microbiome-based therapeutics. These treatments aim to modify the gut microbiome to prevent or cure diseases.

Fecal Microbiota Transplantation (FMT)

One of the most promising areas is fecal microbiota transplantation, where stool from a healthy donor is transplanted into a patient's gut. FMT has been successful in treating Clostridioides difficile infections and is being explored for conditions like IBD, obesity, and type 2 diabetes.

Engineered Probiotics

Another exciting development is the creation of engineered probiotics, where bacteria are genetically modified to treat specific diseases. These could include bacteria designed to produce therapeutic compounds, target pathogenic bacteria, or modulate the immune system.

Personalized Microbiome Interventions

Advancements in personalized medicine are extending to microbiome research, with treatments being tailored to individual microbiome profiles.

Microbiome Testing and Personalized Diets

Personalized diets based on microbiome testing are becoming more common. These diets are designed to promote beneficial bacteria and reduce harmful ones, tailored to an individual's unique microbiome composition.

Targeted Prebiotics

Developing prebiotics that target specific beneficial microbes in the gut is another area of focus. These could be used to selectively nourish and enhance populations of bacteria that are beneficial for specific conditions or overall health.

Pharmacobiomics: Drugs and the Microbiome

Pharmacobiomics, the study of how the microbiome influences drug metabolism, is an emerging field. Understanding the interplay between medications and the microbiome can lead to more effective dosing and reduced side effects.

Microbiome-based Drug Metabolism

Research is revealing that the efficacy and toxicity of certain drugs are influenced by the gut microbiome. In the future, treatments may be adjusted based on an individual's microbiome profile to optimize drug efficacy and minimize adverse effects.

Microbiome and Mental Health

With the growing understanding of the gut-brain axis, the microbiome is being explored as a target for treating mental health disorders.

Psychobiotics

The concept of psychobiotics, or probiotics that have beneficial effects on mental health, is being researched. These could be used to treat conditions like depression, anxiety, and stress-related disorders.

Immune System Modulation

The intricate relationship between the microbiome and the immune system is leading to the development of microbiome-based immunotherapies.

Autoimmune and Inflammatory Diseases

Treatments that modulate the microbiome to influence the immune system are being explored for autoimmune and inflammatory diseases. These therapies aim to restore immune tolerance and reduce inflammation.

Cancer Treatment and the Microbiome

Emerging research suggests that the microbiome may play a role in the effectiveness of cancer treatments.

Microbiome and Chemotherapy

Studies are investigating how the microbiome affects the response to chemotherapy. In the future, modulating the microbiome could become a part of cancer treatment protocols to enhance the effectiveness of chemotherapy.

Microbiome-based Cancer Therapies

There is also interest in developing microbiome-based therapies that could directly target cancer cells or enhance the body's natural immune response to cancer.

Challenges and Future Directions

Despite the exciting potential of microbiome-based therapies, there are challenges and considerations that must be addressed:

Ethical and Regulatory Concerns

The development of microbiome therapies involves navigating complex ethical and regulatory landscapes, particularly concerning genetic modifications and donor material for FMT.

Standardization and Safety

Standardizing microbiome therapies and ensuring their safety and efficacy is crucial. Ongoing clinical trials and research are vital in establishing guidelines and protocols.

Understanding Mechanisms of Action

A deeper understanding of the mechanisms by which the microbiome influences health and disease is essential for the development of effective treatments.

Conclusion

The future of microbiome-based therapies and treatments is incredibly promising, offering potential breakthroughs in a wide range of diseases. From personalized dietary interventions to genetically engineered probiotics and microbiome-influenced drug therapies, the possibilities are vast. As we continue to explore this fascinating frontier, we edge closer to a new era in medicine where the microbiome is a central focus in health and disease management. This burgeoning field not only holds the promise of novel treatments but also underscores the importance of maintaining a healthy microbiome for overall well-being.

Chapter 10: Practical Strategies for Everyday Wellness

Daily Habits for a Healthy Microbiome

The quest for optimal health is intricately linked to the well-being of our gut microbiome. This complex and dynamic community of microorganisms plays a crucial role in various aspects of our health, from digestion and immunity to mental well-being. Cultivating a healthy microbiome is not about quick fixes; it's about integrating mindful daily habits that support these microbial allies. This chapter provides a comprehensive guide to everyday habits that can foster a thriving and balanced gut microbiome.

Embrace a Diverse, Fiber-Rich Diet

The foundation of a healthy microbiome is a varied and nutrient-rich diet. Diversity in the diet translates to diversity in the microbiome, which is key to its resilience and functionality.

Incorporate Various Plant-Based Foods

Eating a wide array of plant-based foods ensures a supply of different types of fibers and phytonutrients, which serve as food for beneficial gut bacteria. Aim to include a variety of fruits, vegetables, legumes, grains, nuts, and seeds in your daily diet.

Focus on High-Fiber Foods

Fiber is particularly crucial for gut health as it is fermented by gut bacteria into beneficial short-chain fatty acids. Foods like whole grains, beans, lentils, berries, and leafy greens are excellent sources of fiber.

Include Fermented Foods in Your Diet

Fermented foods are natural sources of beneficial bacteria and can help augment the diversity of your gut microbiome.

Regularly Consume Probiotic-Rich Foods

Incorporate foods like yogurt, kefir, sauerkraut, kimchi, miso, and kombucha into your diet. These foods provide probiotics that can help balance the gut microbiome.

Stay Hydrated

Adequate hydration is essential for overall health and the well-being of your gut microbiome. Water aids digestion, nutrient absorption, and the elimination of waste, which helps maintain a healthy gut environment.

Drink Plenty of Water

Aim to drink enough water throughout the day to support digestive processes and overall body function.

Manage Stress

Chronic stress can have a detrimental impact on the gut microbiome. Managing stress effectively is thus an important aspect of maintaining gut health.

Practice Stress-Reduction Techniques

Engage in activities like meditation, yoga, deep breathing exercises, or any relaxing hobby that helps in managing stress.

Get Adequate and Quality Sleep

Sleep has a profound impact on gut health, and poor sleep can disrupt the microbiome.

Prioritize Sleep

Ensure 7-9 hours of quality sleep each night. Establish a regular sleep schedule and create a restful sleeping environment.

Regular Physical Activity

Exercise not only benefits overall health but also positively impacts gut microbiome diversity.

Incorporate Moderate Exercise

Regular moderate exercise, such as brisk walking, cycling, or swimming, can enhance the diversity and functionality of the gut microbiome.

Avoid Unnecessary Antibiotics

While antibiotics are necessary for treating certain infections, their overuse can disrupt the gut microbiome.

Use Antibiotics Judiciously

Only take antibiotics when prescribed by a healthcare professional, and always complete the prescribed course.

Limit Alcohol and Avoid Smoking

Excessive alcohol consumption and smoking can have negative effects on gut health.

Practice Moderation

If you consume alcohol, do so in moderation. Avoid smoking, as it can lead to an imbalance in the gut microbiome.

Minimize Intake of Processed Foods

Processed foods, especially those high in sugar and unhealthy fats, can promote the growth of harmful bacteria in the gut.

Opt for Whole, Unprocessed Foods

Choose fresh and minimally processed foods as much as possible. This not only supports the microbiome but also overall health.

Practice Mindful Eating

How you eat can be just as important as what you eat. Mindful eating helps in better digestion and nutrient absorption.

Eat Slowly and Without Distractions

Take time to chew your food thoroughly and eat without distractions like television or smartphones.

Monitor Your Gut Health

Paying attention to your body's signals can help you understand what benefits or harms your gut microbiome.

Keep a Food and Symptom Diary

Tracking what you eat and any digestive symptoms you experience can help identify foods that support or hinder your gut health.

Conclusion

Maintaining a healthy gut microbiome is an ongoing process that involves mindful choices and habits. By focusing on a diverse, fiber-rich diet, managing stress, prioritizing sleep, engaging in regular physical activity, and avoiding harmful substances, you can create an environment where beneficial gut bacteria can thrive. These daily habits not only support a healthy microbiome but also contribute to overall physical and mental well-being. Embracing these practices can lead to a more balanced life and a harmonious relationship with the microscopic world within us.

Recipes for Gut Health

Nurturing a healthy gut microbiome is essential for overall well-being, and one of the most effective ways to do this is through diet. Integrating gut-friendly recipes into your daily meal plan can provide the necessary nutrients to support and maintain a balanced microbiome. This chapter focuses on delicious and nutritious recipes designed to boost gut health, featuring ingredients rich in probiotics, prebiotics, and fiber.

Fermented Oats with Berries and Nuts

Ingredients:

- Rolled oats
- Kefir or Greek yogurt
- Mixed berries (blueberries, strawberries, raspberries)
- Chopped nuts (almonds, walnuts)
- A drizzle of honey or maple syrup (optional)
- Ground flaxseeds or chia seeds

Preparation:

1. Soak the rolled oats in kefir or Greek yogurt overnight in the refrigerator.

2. In the morning, stir the mixture and add more kefir or yogurt if needed to reach your desired consistency.

3. Top with mixed berries, chopped nuts, and a sprinkle of ground flaxseeds or chia seeds.

4. For a touch of sweetness, drizzle with honey or maple syrup.

5. Enjoy this probiotic-rich breakfast that's also packed with fiber and antioxidants.

Hearty Lentil Soup

Ingredients:

- Olive oil
- Diced onions, carrots, and celery
- Minced garlic
- Vegetable or chicken broth
- Brown or green lentils, rinsed
- Diced tomatoes

- Spinach or kale
- Salt, pepper, and herbs (thyme, rosemary)

Preparation:

1. In a large pot, heat olive oil over medium heat and sauté onions, carrots, and celery until soft.

2. Add minced garlic and cook for another minute.

3. Pour in the broth and add lentils. Bring to a boil, then simmer until lentils are tender.

4. Add diced tomatoes and continue to simmer.

5. A few minutes before serving, add spinach or kale and let it wilt.

6. Season with salt, pepper, and herbs.

7. This soup is rich in fiber and nutrients, perfect for supporting gut health.

Grilled Salmon with Quinoa Salad

Ingredients:

- Salmon fillets
- Cooked quinoa
- Mixed salad greens
- Cherry tomatoes, halved
- Cucumber, sliced
- Avocado, sliced
- Olive oil and lemon juice
- Salt and pepper

Preparation:

1. Grill the salmon fillets with a bit of olive oil, salt, and pepper.

2. In a bowl, mix cooked quinoa with salad greens, cherry tomatoes, cucumber, and avocado.

3. Dress the salad with olive oil and lemon juice, and season with salt and pepper.

4. Serve the salad with the grilled salmon on top.

5. This meal is rich in omega-3 fatty acids, fiber, and probiotics, making it excellent for gut health.

Roasted Vegetable and Hummus Wrap

Ingredients:

- Whole grain tortillas
- Hummus
- Assorted vegetables (bell peppers, zucchini, eggplant)
- Olive oil
- Salt and pepper
- Mixed greens or spinach

Preparation:

1. Slice the vegetables and roast them in the oven with olive oil, salt, and pepper until tender.

2. Spread hummus on whole grain tortillas.

3. Place a layer of mixed greens or spinach on top of the hummus.

4. Add the roasted vegetables to the tortillas.

5. Roll the tortillas into wraps.

6. These wraps are a great source of fiber and plant-based protein, promoting a healthy gut.

Berry and Yogurt Smoothie

Ingredients:

- Mixed berries (fresh or frozen)
- Plain Greek yogurt or kefir
- Banana
- Almond milk or milk of choice
- A scoop of protein powder (optional)
- Honey or maple syrup (optional)

Preparation:

1. Blend mixed berries, Greek yogurt or kefir, banana, and almond milk until smooth.

2. Add protein powder if using, and sweeten with honey or maple syrup if desired.

3. This smoothie is not only delicious but also packed with probiotics and antioxidants, making it a gut health powerhouse.

Conclusion

These recipes are not only delicious but also packed with gut-friendly ingredients. Regularly incorporating such meals into your diet can significantly contribute to a healthy and balanced gut microbiome. Remember, the key to gut health is diversity – a variety of foods ensures a variety of nutrients, fostering a thriving microbial community. Enjoy these recipes as part of your journey towards better gut health and overall wellness.

Mindful Practices for Microbial Balance

In the pursuit of a healthy gut microbiome, the importance of mindfulness and intentional living cannot be overstated. Beyond diet and physical activity, our mental and emotional states play a significant role in maintaining microbial balance. This chapter delves into various mindful practices that can positively influence the gut microbiome, highlighting the interconnectedness of mental, emotional, and gut health.

The Gut-Brain Connection and Mindfulness

The gut-brain axis, a complex communication network that links the gastrointestinal system with the brain, is significantly influenced by our mental and emotional states. Stress, anxiety, and emotional turmoil can disrupt this delicate balance, leading to changes in gut microbiome composition and function. Mindful practices can mitigate these effects, promoting a sense of calm and balance that is conducive to a healthy gut.

Stress Reduction Techniques

Meditation and Deep Breathing

Meditation and deep breathing exercises are effective in reducing stress and promoting relaxation. Regular practice can lower cortisol levels, a stress hormone that can negatively impact gut health. Mindfulness meditation, in particular, encourages a state of awareness and presence, helping to manage stress and its physiological impacts.

Yoga

Yoga, which combines physical postures, breath control, and meditation, is another powerful tool for stress reduction. It not only helps in reducing stress but also improves physical health, both of which are beneficial for the gut microbiome.

Quality Sleep for Gut Health

Establishing a Sleep Routine

Adequate and quality sleep is vital for maintaining a healthy gut microbiome. Poor sleep can disrupt the gut-brain axis and lead to imbalances in gut bacteria. Establishing a regular sleep routine, ensuring a comfortable sleep environment, and avoiding stimulants like caffeine and electronics before bedtime can improve sleep quality.

Relaxation Techniques Before Bed

Practices such as reading, taking a warm bath, or gentle stretching can promote relaxation and improve the quality of sleep, positively affecting gut health.

Mindful Eating for Gut Wellness

Eating Without Distractions

Mindful eating involves being fully present during meals, eating slowly, and paying attention to the sensations and experiences associated with eating. Eating without distractions like TV or smartphones allows for better digestion and can prevent overeating, which is beneficial for the gut.

Listening to the Body's Signals

Paying attention to hunger and fullness cues and noticing how different foods affect your body can help in identifying foods that support or hinder gut health.

Emotional Wellness and Gut Health

Emotional Expression and Processing

Emotional health is closely tied to gut health. Practices that promote emotional expression and processing, such as journaling, talking to a trusted friend or therapist, and engaging in creative activities, can help maintain a balanced gut microbiome.

Gratitude and Positive Thinking

Cultivating gratitude and positive thinking can improve mental health and, in turn, support gut health. Keeping a gratitude journal or regularly reflecting on positive aspects of life can have beneficial effects on the gut-brain axis.

Connection with Nature

Spending Time Outdoors

Regular exposure to natural environments can enhance the diversity of the microbiome. Activities like hiking, gardening, or simply spending time in a park can introduce beneficial microbes and reduce stress.

Regular Physical Activity

Mindful Movement

Engaging in physical activities that you enjoy and are mindful, such as walking, swimming, or dancing, can improve gut health. Exercise not only reduces stress but also directly impacts the composition and diversity of the gut microbiome.

Limiting Alcohol and Quitting Smoking

Mindfulness in Lifestyle Choices

Being mindful of the impact of alcohol and smoking on the gut is important. Limiting alcohol consumption and quitting smoking can prevent negative effects on the gut microbiome and contribute to overall health.

Community and Social Connections

Building Healthy Relationships

Social interactions and a sense of community can positively impact mental and emotional health, which in turn can benefit the gut microbiome. Engaging in social activities, connecting with loved ones, and being part of a community can promote a balanced gut.

Conclusion

Cultivating a healthy gut microbiome goes beyond dietary and physical habits; it encompasses a holistic approach that includes mindful practices. By integrating stress reduction techniques, quality sleep, mindful eating, emotional wellness practices, and a connection with nature and community into our daily lives, we can support our gut microbiome. These practices not only enhance our microbial balance but also contribute to overall health and well-being, underscoring the importance of a comprehensive approach to wellness. As we continue to learn about the profound connections between our mind, body, and gut, adopting mindful practices becomes an essential part of nurturing our health.

Chapter 11:
The Future of Microbiome Health

Predictions and Trends in Microbiome Research

The exploration of the human microbiome, one of the most vibrant and rapidly evolving fields in contemporary science, holds immense promise for the future of healthcare and wellness. As researchers delve deeper into the complexities of the gut microbiome, new predictions and trends are emerging, offering exciting glimpses into the potential applications and advancements we may see in the coming years. This chapter explores these predictions and trends, highlighting how they could shape our understanding of health and disease.

Personalized Microbiome Healthcare

One of the most significant trends in microbiome research is the shift towards personalized healthcare. As we understand more about how individual microbiome profiles can influence health, personalized dietary recommendations, probiotic supplements, and treatments become more targeted and effective.

Tailored Dietary Plans

Future dietary guidelines may be customized based on one's microbiome profile, leading to more effective nutrition strategies for health and disease prevention.

Customized Probiotics and Prebiotics

We are likely to see the development of probiotics and prebiotics tailored to the needs of an individual's specific gut flora, enhancing the effectiveness of these supplements.

Advances in Microbiome Testing

The field of microbiome testing is rapidly advancing, with newer, more sophisticated technologies providing detailed insights into the gut flora.

Non-Invasive Diagnostics

Emerging diagnostic tools, which are less invasive and more comprehensive, will enable regular monitoring of gut health and early detection of imbalances or diseases.

Real-Time Microbiome Analysis

Future advancements may allow for real-time monitoring of the gut microbiome, providing immediate feedback on the impact of diet, lifestyle, and medication.

Microbiome and Mental Health

The gut-brain axis is a key area of exploration, with significant implications for mental health.

Microbiome-based Treatments for Mental Disorders

Predictions include the development of microbiome-based therapies for conditions like depression, anxiety, and even neurodegenerative diseases.

Stress and Gut Health

More research is likely to focus on how stress management and relaxation techniques can beneficially modify the gut microbiome.

Microbiome and Chronic Diseases

The link between the microbiome and chronic diseases such as obesity, diabetes, and heart disease is a growing area of research.

Predictive Microbiome Profiling

Researchers may soon be able to predict an individual's risk of developing certain chronic diseases based on their microbiome profile.

Microbiome Modulation as Therapy

Future therapies may include microbiome modulation as a standard treatment for various chronic conditions.

Environmental Influences on the Microbiome

The impact of environmental factors on the microbiome is becoming increasingly apparent, guiding new approaches in public health and policy.

Urban Planning and Microbiome Health

There may be a growing emphasis on urban planning and environmental policies that consider the impact on the microbiome, such as reducing pollution and increasing green spaces.

Microbiome-Friendly Lifestyle Guidelines

Guidelines and recommendations for maintaining a healthy microbiome, including exposure to diverse environments and reducing chemical exposures, may become common.

Advances in Microbiome-Gut-Brain Axis Research

The interplay between the gut microbiome and the brain is a rapidly expanding field, with significant implications for neurological health.

Neurological Disorders and the Microbiome

Research is expected to delve deeper into how the gut microbiome influences conditions like Alzheimer's, Parkinson's, and autism spectrum disorders.

Gut Health and Cognitive Function

Studies may increasingly focus on how maintaining a healthy gut can positively affect cognitive function and mental clarity.

The Future of Probiotics and Synbiotics

Innovations in probiotic and synbiotic formulations are anticipated, with a focus on increased efficacy and targeted actions.

Next-Generation Probiotics

Future probiotics may include strains of bacteria specifically engineered to treat or prevent specific diseases.

Enhanced Synbiotic Products

Synbiotics, which combine probiotics and prebiotics, are likely to become more sophisticated, offering tailored combinations for optimal gut health.

Conclusion

The future of microbiome research is bright and filled with possibilities. As we continue to unravel the mysteries of the gut microbiome, its profound impact on health and disease becomes increasingly evident. Personalized microbiome healthcare, advanced testing methods, a deeper understanding of the microbiome's role in mental and chronic diseases, and the development of new probiotic and synbiotic formulations are just a few of the exciting trends on the horizon. These advancements promise not only a better understanding of human biology but also a new era in healthcare, where maintaining and restoring microbiome balance is central to preventing and treating a wide range of conditions. The future of microbiome health is poised to be an integral part of holistic health and wellness, emphasizing the importance of nurturing our microbial allies for optimal health.

The Expanding Role of Gut Health in Medicine

The significance of gut health in the realm of medicine is undergoing a transformative shift. With the burgeoning research on the human microbiome, the medical community is increasingly recognizing the gut's critical role in overall health and disease prevention. This chapter explores the expanding role of gut health in medicine, discussing how emerging research and developments are reshaping healthcare practices and offering new therapeutic possibilities.

Gut Microbiome as a Pillar of Health

The gut microbiome is now considered a pivotal component of human health, akin to an organ system in its complexity and importance. Its influence extends beyond digestion, impacting immune function, mental health, and chronic disease risk.

A Holistic View of Health

The medical community is increasingly adopting a holistic view of health, acknowledging the interconnectedness of the gut microbiome with various bodily systems. This perspective fosters a more comprehensive approach to health and disease management.

Preventive Healthcare

Understanding the role of the gut in disease prevention is leading to a greater emphasis on preventive healthcare. Proactive measures to maintain a balanced gut microbiome are being recognized as crucial steps in preventing a wide array of health issues.

Diagnostic and Therapeutic Advances

Advancements in understanding the gut microbiome are driving innovations in diagnostics and therapeutics.

Microbiome Profiling in Diagnostics

The use of microbiome profiling as a diagnostic tool is an emerging trend. Analyzing the composition of the gut microbiome can aid in diagnosing various conditions, from gastrointestinal disorders to metabolic diseases and even mental health issues.

Microbiome-Based Therapeutics

The development of microbiome-based therapies, such as customized probiotics, prebiotics, and fecal microbiota transplants (FMT), is a rapidly growing area. These therapies aim to restore or modify the gut microbiome to treat or manage diseases.

The Gut-Brain Axis in Psychiatry

The understanding of the gut-brain axis is revolutionizing the field of psychiatry. The link between gut health and mental health opens new avenues for treating psychiatric disorders.

Psychobiotics

The concept of psychobiotics, probiotics that can improve mental health, is gaining traction. These may become integral in treating conditions like depression, anxiety, and stress-related disorders.

Integrative Approaches to Mental Health

There is a growing recognition of the need for integrative approaches in psychiatry, incorporating gut health strategies alongside traditional psychological therapies.

Personalized Nutrition

Personalized nutrition, tailored to an individual's unique gut microbiome, is becoming a key focus in healthcare.

Diet as a Therapeutic Tool

Dietary recommendations based on microbiome analysis can be used as a therapeutic tool, personalized to improve specific health outcomes.

The Role of Dietitians and Nutritionists

Dietitians and nutritionists are playing an increasingly important role in healthcare teams, providing expertise in devising diet plans that support gut health and overall well-being.

Impact on Autoimmune and Inflammatory Diseases

The link between the gut microbiome and the immune system is providing new insights into autoimmune and inflammatory diseases.

Targeting the Microbiome in Autoimmunity

Targeting the gut microbiome is emerging as a strategy in managing autoimmune conditions, such as rheumatoid arthritis and type 1 diabetes.

Anti-Inflammatory Diets

The adoption of anti-inflammatory diets, which support a healthy gut microbiome, is being recognized as an effective approach in reducing chronic inflammation and managing inflammatory diseases.

Challenges and Future Directions

While the expanding role of gut health in medicine offers exciting possibilities, it also presents challenges.

Need for Further Research

Further research is needed to fully understand the complex interactions within the gut microbiome and how they impact health and disease.

Integrating New Knowledge into Practice

Integrating this rapidly evolving knowledge into clinical practice is a challenge. Ongoing education and training for healthcare professionals are essential.

Ethical and Regulatory Considerations

The development of microbiome-based therapies involves navigating ethical and regulatory considerations, particularly regarding the use of genetic information and donor material for FMT.

Conclusion

The expanding role of gut health in medicine is a testament to the dynamic nature of medical science and its responsiveness to new research. As we continue to uncover the complexities and vast influence of the gut microbiome, its integration into medical practice is becoming increasingly vital. From diagnostics and treatment to preventive healthcare and nutrition, the focus on gut health is set to transform the landscape of medicine. This shift not only promises more effective and personalized care but also underscores the importance of a holistic approach to health, where the gut microbiome is recognized as a central factor in maintaining overall well-being. As research continues to advance, the future of medicine will undoubtedly see the gut microbiome playing a key role in shaping health outcomes and therapeutic strategies.

The Next Frontier in Microbiome Wellness

As we venture further into the 21st century, the exploration of the human microbiome stands at the forefront of a new era in health and wellness. The vast and intricate universe of microorganisms residing within us is increasingly recognized as a key player in our overall well-being, with the potential to transform how we approach health, disease prevention, and treatment. This chapter discusses the next frontier in microbiome wellness, examining the emerging trends, potential breakthroughs, and innovative approaches that could redefine our understanding of health in the years to come.

Personalized Microbiome Management

The future of microbiome wellness lies in the realm of personalization. As we gather more detailed and sophisticated data on individual microbiome profiles, we move closer to personalized microbiome management, which tailors dietary, lifestyle, and medical interventions to an individual's specific microbiome makeup.

Tailored Dietary Recommendations

Nutritional plans based on one's unique microbiome composition could optimize gut health, enhance metabolic efficiency, and reduce the risk of various diseases.

Customized Probiotics and Prebiotics

Advances in biotechnology may enable the creation of probiotics and prebiotics designed to target specific imbalances in an individual's microbiome, offering more effective and personalized approaches to gut health.

Breakthroughs in Microbiome Therapeutics

The therapeutic potential of the microbiome is vast, with research increasingly focusing on harnessing this potential to treat a wide range of conditions.

Microbiome-based Disease Treatment

Future therapies may include microbiome manipulation as a standard treatment for diseases ranging from gastrointestinal disorders to metabolic conditions, autoimmune diseases, and even mental health issues.

Fecal Microbiota Transplantation (FMT) Expansion

The application of FMT could expand beyond Clostridioides difficile infections, potentially offering solutions for a variety of health issues linked to microbiome imbalances.

The Gut-Brain Axis and Mental Health

The gut-brain axis is likely to become a major focus in both research and treatment strategies, particularly in the field of mental health.

Microbiome's Role in Neurological and Psychiatric Disorders

Further understanding of how the gut microbiome influences brain function could lead to breakthroughs in treating neurological and psychiatric disorders.

Stress Management and Emotional Wellbeing

Innovative approaches may emerge focusing on how modulation of the gut microbiome can aid in stress management and promote emotional wellbeing.

Technological Advancements in Microbiome Research

Technological innovation is set to revolutionize microbiome research, offering new tools and methodologies for understanding and manipulating this complex ecosystem.

Advanced Genomic Sequencing Techniques

These techniques will provide deeper insights into the composition and function of the microbiome, paving the way for novel interventions and therapies.

Artificial Intelligence and Machine Learning

AI and machine learning could be used to analyze large datasets, predict microbiome-related health outcomes, and personalize treatment strategies.

Environmental and Lifestyle Factors

As we recognize the impact of environmental and lifestyle factors on the microbiome, there will be a shift towards creating more microbiome-friendly environments and lifestyles.

Urban Planning and Public Health Policies

Future urban planning and public health policies may incorporate considerations for microbiome health, such as reducing pollution and increasing green spaces.

Lifestyle Interventions

Emphasis on lifestyle interventions that support microbiome health, including stress reduction, sleep optimization, and regular physical activity, will likely increase.

Integrative and Holistic Approaches

The future of microbiome wellness will likely embrace more integrative and holistic approaches, combining traditional medicine with alternative therapies to support gut health.

Combining Conventional and Alternative Therapies

Integrating dietary interventions, lifestyle changes, and conventional medical treatments could provide a more comprehensive approach to managing and improving gut health.

Education and Public Awareness

As the importance of the microbiome becomes more widely recognized, there will likely be a greater emphasis on education and public awareness.

Microbiome Literacy

Educational initiatives could focus on increasing microbiome literacy, helping individuals understand the importance of gut health and how to support it.

Challenges and Ethical Considerations

With these advancements come challenges and ethical considerations, particularly regarding data privacy, the commercialization of microbiome information, and ensuring equitable access to emerging treatments and technologies.

Conclusion

The next frontier in microbiome wellness is ripe with possibilities, offering exciting prospects for health and disease management. Personalized microbiome management, breakthroughs in therapeutics, technological advancements, and an integrative approach to health and wellness are just some of the trends that could shape the future landscape of microbiome wellness. As we continue to explore and understand this complex ecosystem within us, our approach to health and disease is poised for transformation, promising a future where the maintenance and enhancement of microbiome health are central to achieving overall well-being.

Chapter 12: Conclusion

Summarizing the Power of Gut Instincts

As we reach the conclusion of this exploration into the fascinating world of the gut microbiome, it's clear that the phrase 'gut instincts' encompasses much more than an intuitive feeling. It represents the intricate and profound influence of our gut microbiome on our overall health and well-being. This chapter summarizes the key insights gleaned from our journey through the complex and dynamic universe of the gut microbiome, highlighting its critical role in various aspects of our lives.

The Gut Microbiome: A Central Pillar of Health

The gut microbiome, a diverse community of microorganisms residing in our gastrointestinal tract, has emerged as a central pillar of health. It plays a crucial role in digestion, nutrient absorption, immune function, and even impacts our mental health through the gut-brain axis. The balance and diversity of this microbial ecosystem are essential for maintaining optimal health, and disruptions to this balance can lead to a myriad of health issues.

Diet and the Microbiome

Our exploration underscored the profound impact of diet on the gut microbiome. A diet rich in diverse, fiber-rich foods fosters a healthy microbiome, enhancing its diversity and functionality. Incorporating fermented foods and probiotics into our diet supports the growth of beneficial bacteria, while limiting processed foods and excessive sugars helps prevent microbial imbalances. The intimate connection between what we eat and our gut health highlights the importance of mindful eating for maintaining a balanced microbiome.

Lifestyle and Environmental Influences

Lifestyle factors, including stress management, quality sleep, and regular exercise, play significant roles in shaping our gut microbiome. Chronic stress, poor sleep, and a sedentary lifestyle can negatively impact microbial balance, emphasizing the need for holistic approaches to health that consider both physical and mental well-being. Environmental factors, such as exposure to pollutants and antibiotics, also influence the microbiome, guiding us towards more conscious choices about our surroundings and their impact on our health.

The Gut-Brain Axis and Mental Health

The gut-brain axis has emerged as a key area of interest, revealing the complex interactions between the gut microbiome and our mental health. The microbiome's role in producing neurotransmitters, modulating inflammation, and interacting with the nervous system opens new avenues for understanding and treating mental health disorders. This connection underscores the potential of targeting the gut microbiome in strategies for mental wellness.

Therapeutic Potential of the Microbiome

The therapeutic potential of the microbiome is vast, with emerging treatments like fecal microbiota transplantation and customized probiotics offering new hope for various health conditions. The development of microbiome-based therapies for diseases such as inflammatory bowel diseases, obesity, and even certain types of cancer illustrates the microbiome's critical role in medicine's future.

Personalized Microbiome Healthcare

The trend towards personalized microbiome healthcare, where treatments and dietary recommendations are tailored to an individual's unique microbiome profile, represents a significant shift in medical practice. This approach promises more effective and personalized care, emphasizing the importance of understanding and nurturing our individual microbiome for optimal health.

The Future of Microbiome Research

Looking forward, microbiome research is poised to continue transforming our understanding of health and disease. Advances in technology and a deeper understanding of the microbiome's complexities will likely lead to novel diagnostic tools, more targeted treatments, and a greater emphasis on preventive health measures that support a healthy gut.

Education and Public Awareness

As public awareness of the microbiome's importance grows, so does the need for education and literacy in this field. Understanding how to support and maintain a healthy gut microbiome will become increasingly important, guiding individuals in making informed choices about their diet, lifestyle, and healthcare.

Ethical and Global Considerations

Finally, the exploration of the gut microbiome raises ethical and global considerations, from data privacy in microbiome testing to ensuring equitable access to emerging treatments and technologies. As we venture further into this field, it is crucial to navigate these challenges thoughtfully and responsibly.

Conclusion

In summarizing the power of gut instincts, we recognize the gut microbiome as a key determinant of our health and a reflection of our lifestyle and environmental interactions. The journey through the world of the gut microbiome highlights the profound impact of this hidden universe within us. It's a testament to the intricate connections that govern our body and health, emphasizing the importance of nurturing our gut microbiome for overall well-being. As we continue to uncover the mysteries of the gut, we are reminded of the wisdom embedded in our 'gut instincts,' guiding us towards a healthier, more balanced life.

The Continuous Journey of Microbial Health

As we conclude our exploration of the human microbiome, it becomes evident that caring for our microbial health is a continuous journey, not a destination. This intricate ecosystem within us plays a fundamental role in our overall health and well-being, influencing everything from our digestive processes to our immune system and even our mental health. This chapter reflects on the journey of microbial health, underscoring its ongoing nature and the dynamic interplay between our lifestyle, environment, and the microscopic world within us.

Understanding the Dynamic Nature of the Microbiome

The human microbiome is not a static entity; it is a vibrant and ever-changing ecosystem. Factors such as diet, lifestyle, age, and environment continuously shape its composition and functionality. Recognizing this dynamic nature is crucial in appreciating that maintaining a healthy microbiome is an ongoing process, requiring consistent attention and care.

The Impact of Diet and Lifestyle

Our dietary choices and lifestyle habits have immediate and long-term effects on our microbiome. A diet rich in diverse, whole foods supports a balanced microbiome, while processed foods and a sedentary lifestyle can lead to imbalances. Regular physical activity, stress management, and adequate sleep are equally important in maintaining microbial health.

The Role of the Microbiome in Disease Prevention

The gut microbiome plays a critical role in disease prevention. A balanced microbiome can strengthen the immune system, reduce inflammation, and lower the risk of various chronic diseases. This preventive aspect underscores the importance of ongoing efforts to nurture our microbiome as part of a holistic approach to health.

Personalized Approaches to Disease Prevention

As we learn more about the microbiome, personalized approaches to disease prevention are becoming more prevalent. Understanding individual microbiome profiles can guide tailored dietary and lifestyle interventions, enhancing their effectiveness in preventing disease.

The Interconnectedness of Gut Health and Mental Well-being

The gut-brain axis highlights the interconnectedness of our gut health and mental well-being. The microbiome's influence on mood, stress response, and cognitive function demonstrates that caring for our gut is also caring for our mind.

Mindfulness and Gut Health

Incorporating mindfulness practices like meditation and yoga can positively affect the gut-brain axis, offering a holistic approach to maintaining mental and microbial health.

Advances in Microbiome Research

The field of microbiome research is continuously evolving, bringing new insights and innovations. These advances are not only enhancing our understanding of the microbiome but also opening up new possibilities for treatments and therapies.

The Future of Microbiome-Based Therapies

Emerging microbiome-based therapies, such as tailored probiotics and fecal microbiota transplantation, are promising areas of research. As these therapies develop, they could offer more effective and personalized solutions for various health conditions.

The Global Perspective on Microbial Health

Microbial health is not just an individual concern; it's a global one. Factors such as diet trends, environmental changes, and the use of antibiotics have global implications for microbial health.

Addressing Global Challenges

Addressing the challenges facing microbial health, such as antibiotic resistance and the impact of environmental pollutants, requires a collective effort. Global initiatives and policies that promote microbial health are essential.

Education and Public Awareness

Raising public awareness and education about the importance of microbial health is vital. As people become more knowledgeable about the role of the microbiome, they can make informed decisions about their diet, lifestyle, and healthcare.

The Role of Healthcare Professionals

Healthcare professionals play a crucial role in educating patients about microbial health and integrating microbiome considerations into clinical practice.

The Journey of Self-Discovery and Health

Understanding and nurturing our microbiome is also a journey of self-discovery. It encourages us to listen to our bodies, understand our unique health needs, and make mindful choices that support our well-being.

Personalized Health Journeys

Each individual's journey to microbial health will be different, guided by their unique microbiome, lifestyle, and health goals. Embracing this personalized journey is key to achieving optimal health.

Conclusion

The journey of microbial health is a continuous one, requiring ongoing effort, adaptability, and a holistic perspective. As we navigate this journey, we are guided by the latest research, mindful practices, and an understanding of our unique health needs. By embracing the dynamic nature of our microbiome and the interconnectedness of our overall health, we can make choices that nurture our microbial allies and, in turn, our entire being. The journey of microbial health is not just about preventing disease or addressing health issues; it's about cultivating vitality, resilience, and well-being for a lifetime.

Empowering Readers to Take Control of Their Gut Health

In the journey towards achieving optimal health, understanding and nurturing our gut microbiome emerges as a key element. This concluding chapter aims to empower readers with the knowledge and tools necessary to take control of their gut health. By embracing the insights gained from the intricate world of microbiomes, we can make informed decisions that positively impact our overall well-being.

The Foundation of Gut Health

Understanding the Microbiome's Influence

Recognizing the gut microbiome's influence on various aspects of health – from digestion and immunity to mental well-being – is the first step in taking control. A balanced microbiome supports efficient digestion, robust immune defense, and even balanced mental health through the gut-brain axis.

The Role of Diet and Nutrition

Diet plays a pivotal role in shaping the gut microbiome. Incorporating a diverse range of nutrient-rich foods, especially those high in fiber, can foster a healthy and diverse microbial community. Regularly consuming fermented foods like yogurt, kefir, and sauerkraut can introduce beneficial bacteria to the gut.

Lifestyle Factors Affecting Gut Health

Stress Management

Stress can have a significant impact on the gut microbiome. Engaging in stress-reduction techniques such as meditation, yoga, or even simple deep-breathing exercises can mitigate these effects and promote gut health.

Importance of Physical Activity

Regular physical activity is not only beneficial for overall health but also positively influences the gut microbiome. Even moderate activities like walking can enhance microbial diversity and functionality.

Prioritizing Sleep

Quality sleep is crucial for maintaining a healthy gut microbiome. Establishing a consistent sleep routine and creating a conducive sleep environment are essential steps in this process.

Empowering Through Knowledge

Education on Gut Health

Empowerment comes from understanding. Educating oneself about the intricacies of the gut microbiome and its impact on health enables informed decisions about diet, lifestyle, and medical care.

Keeping Abreast of Research

The field of microbiome research is rapidly evolving. Staying updated on the latest research and scientific discoveries can provide valuable insights into maintaining and improving gut health.

Proactive Health Strategies

Regular Health Check-Ups

Regular consultations with healthcare providers, including discussions about gut health, are essential. Health professionals can offer guidance tailored to individual health needs and conditions.

Mindful Eating Habits

Adopting mindful eating practices – eating slowly, savoring food, and being attentive to hunger and fullness cues – can enhance digestion and gut health.

The Role of Probiotics and Prebiotics

Incorporating Probiotics and Prebiotics

Understanding the role of probiotics and prebiotics in supporting gut health and knowing how to incorporate them into the diet is crucial. This includes choosing the right supplements and consuming foods rich in these beneficial compounds.

Understanding Personalized Gut Health

Individual Variations in Microbiome

Every individual's microbiome is unique. Recognizing this individuality is important in personalizing dietary and lifestyle choices to support one's specific gut health needs.

Personalized Nutrition and Lifestyle Changes

Considering personal health history, preferences, and lifestyle, personalized nutrition plans and lifestyle modifications can be more effective in maintaining optimal gut health.

Community and Support

Building a Supportive Environment

Creating a supportive environment, including family, friends, and community, can provide encouragement and motivation in maintaining gut health. Sharing meals, recipes, and wellness activities can reinforce healthy habits.

Leveraging Online Resources and Communities

Utilizing online resources and communities for information, inspiration, and support can be valuable. Online forums, blogs, and social media groups focused on gut health can provide helpful insights and encouragement.

Addressing Challenges and Setbacks

Overcoming Obstacles

Encountering challenges in maintaining gut health is normal. Developing strategies to overcome these obstacles, such as planning meals, preparing healthy snacks, and finding stress-reduction techniques that work, is key.

Learning from Setbacks

Viewing setbacks as learning opportunities rather than failures can foster resilience and persistence in the journey towards optimal gut health.

Conclusion

Empowering oneself to take control of gut health is an ongoing process that involves education, mindful choices, and lifestyle adjustments. By understanding the profound impact of the gut microbiome on overall health and implementing strategies to nurture it, individuals can enhance their well-being and vitality. This empowerment is not just about preventing or addressing health issues; it's about embracing a lifestyle that supports and sustains a healthy and balanced microbiome. As we close this exploration, the message is clear: taking control of your gut health is a significant step towards achieving a healthier, more balanced life.

www.ingramcontent.com/pod-product-compliance
Lightning Source LLC
Chambersburg PA
CBHW070848260726

48661CB00004B/1311